Excerpts from
The MEDICAL and NUTRITIONAL APPROACH To CANCER

The very word ... **CANCER** ... seems to polarize people into two separate and distinct camps. There is **orthodox medicine.** Most who take this position feel that only orthodox, tested methods are valid. They term anything that doesn't have their approval as *"quackery."* Then, there are the **nutritionists.** Chapter 1

* * *

Cancer has many definitions and many causes. There are three major orthodox treatments for Cancer: Chemotherapy, Surgery, Radiotherapy. Chapter 3

* * *

Five basic drug approaches are used in Chemotherapy. Common side effects are loss of appetite, nausea and hair loss. Impotence can also occur. Chapter 5

* * *

Men have a higher incidence of Colon Cancer. After 40 many men suffer from Cancer of the Prostate. Chapter 8

* * *

Breast Cancer can change marital relationships. The experience will either draw a couple closer together or disrupt the marriage.
Chapter 10

* * *

It is believed Vitamin A interferes and blocks the formation of cancer cells within the body. Carrots have the highest ratio of Vitamin A.
Chapter 12

* * *

Nutritionists suggest that death begins in the colon. They believe a series of colonic irrigations can benefit a cancer sufferer. Knowing one's mineral balance through a hair analysis may provide sensible solutions to illness. Chapter 13

* * *

Sprouts, Wheat Grass and Asparagus are believed by many to be both a cancer preventitive and a possible answer to those with cancer.
Chapter 14

* * *

Visualization Therapy through mental imagery has been successful in healing some patients, according to reports. Chapter 15

* * *

All this and much more you will find in the chapters of this revealing book on *The Medical Approach versus The Nutritional Approach To Cancer!*

Important Legal Notice

Salem Kirban nor Salem Kirban, Inc. does NOT endorse or in any way recommend the data given in this book.

Salem Kirban and Salem Kirban, Inc. acts only as a forum for the presentation of various viewpoints of different individuals, and we do not necessarily agree or disagree with the data published.

The Medical Approach versus The Nutritional Approach series is published for informational and educational purposes only.

If any person decides to follow any data found in this book, the decision rests completely with that person and his doctor, and with no one else. Furthermore, any action or decision taken by any reader concerning which therapies to follow or not to follow, rests, once again, solely with that reader and their doctor. It has nothing to do with Salem Kirban nor Salem Kirban, Inc. or with any employee or agent thereof.

This book is not a substitute for personal medical supervision. No change in diet should ever be made without consultation with your doctor. People with health problems should see their physician.

The Medical Approach
versus
The Nutritional Approach
To
CANCER

by Salem Kirban

Published by SALEM KIRBAN, Inc., Kent Road, Huntingdon Valley, Pennsylvania 19006. Copyright © 1982 by Salem Kirban. Printed in United States of America. All rights reserved, including the right to reproduce this book or portions thereof in any form.

Library of Congress Catalog Card No. 81-84438
ISBN 0-912582-44-8

ACKNOWLEDGMENTS

To **Estelle Bair Composition** for excellence in typesetting.

To **Walter W. Slotilock,** Chapel Hill Litho, for negatives.

To **Bob Jackson,** for medical illustrations on pages 46, 56.

To **Dickinson Brothers, Inc.,** for printing this book.

And special thanks to the following publishers for graciously making available medical illustrations for this book:

Intermed Communications, Inc., Springhouse, Pennsylvania 19477
Illustrations reprinted with permission from <u>Diseases,</u> Copyright © 1981.

J.B. Lippincott Company, Philadelphia, Pennsylvania 19105
Illustrations reprinted with permission from <u>Textbook of Medical-Surgical Nursing</u> by L. Brunner and D. Suddarth, ed. 4, Copyright © 1980.

Mitchell Beazley Publishers, Ltd., England
<u>Atlas of the Body and Mind,</u> Copyright © Mitchell Beazley Publishers, Ltd. 1976. Published in U.S.A. by **Rand McNally & Company.**

Sally Galbraith Thomas, R.N., Ph.D., School of Nursing, University of California for permission to use photographs on pages 58, 66.

CONTENTS

Special Features Include

Over $1 in every $10 Americans spend annually . . . goes for health care. More than $20 Billion each year is spent on Cancer. Cancer is big business. The typical patient spends over $25,000 to treat his or her condition.

Currently over 1 million Americans are under conventional treatment for Cancer. A Cancer patient treated by conventional methods overall has a one-in-three chance of surviving for five years. This is exactly the same odds that faced a Cancer patient in 1950.

When a person is told he has Cancer . . . he is besieged on all sides with conflicting advice. Most likely his doctor and radiologist will strongly advise surgery, radiation or chemotherapy . . . or all three. Friends and loved ones may just as strongly advise alternative approaches. The person with Cancer ultimately must make his own decision. The first step begins with intensive research into understanding your disease.

1

CANCER . . . THE PRICE WE PAY FOR PROGRESS

**Highly
Controversial**

When one writes about Cancer, one deals with perhaps the most controversial subject on health.

The very word . . . **CANCER** . . . seems to polarize people into two separate and distinct camps. There is **orthodox medicine** and most who take this position feel that only orthodox, tested methods are valid. They term anything that doesn't have their approval as "*quackery.*" And some of it is! There are those who prey on the misfortunes of others in both orthodox and unorthodox medicine! Cancer offers them an excellent field to make their fortune!

Then, there are the **nutritionists** who believe that most illness is an indication that the body is lacking certain nutrients . . . and that the supplying of those nutrients is beneficial to restoration to good health.

Most nutritionists feel that drugs, rather than healing, actually interfere with the healing program.

In fact, perhaps more time and money is spent by these two groups in calling each other *"a racket and a fraud"* while those that suffer from Cancer become pawns in a bitter struggle.

Time To Grow Up!

It will be a wonderful day when both orthodox medicine and nutritionists realize neither of them has the final answer to Cancer . . . but that we should all work together. Instead of powerful AMA lobbying, lawsuits and counter-lawsuits . . . it is time we grow up and stop fighting like little children who want sole possession of their little toy.

God made man in His image (Genesis 9:6). And in Psalm 139:14 we are told to praise God:

*For I am fearfully
and wonderfully made!*

Whether we believe in treating Cancer with drugs . . . engrossed in microscopic tests and mountains of data . . . **or** whether we believe in treating Cancer with nutritional therapy . . . we must realize that there is very little we really know not only about Cancer but also about the human body. We may think we have all the answers but the climbing death rate from Cancer should sober us to reality.

**Not A
Single
Disease**

Cancer is not a single disease but a family of disorders. The word Cancer means *crab*. The three basic types of Cancers are:

Carcinoma *Malignant tumor*

Sarcoma   *Cancer arising from underlying tissue: muscle, bone, etc.*

Myeloma *Leukemia and lymphatic disease*

Cancer has been termed: "The body's malignant mystery." The problem is that there are many Cancers ... not one Cancer. There are causes, not one cause.

Some believe that Cancer is a disease of our progressive contemporary society. And there is much truth to this. In the United States we have a high incidence of breast, lung and colon Cancer. In Japan, stomach Cancer is high. And why is it that Uterus Cancer deaths are highest in Pennsylvania, Ohio, Vermont, New Hampshire, Indiana, Illinois, Alabama and South Dakota and lowest in the Western states?

**Emphasis
Misdirected**

One of the complaints lodged against the medical profession is that medical care focuses on disease and ignores health. Whether this is a valid accusation or not, most agree that Cancer will continue to be the second-ranking fatal disease in America surpassed only by Heart Disease.

No one has the complete answer to cancer! Some claim to have been healed of this disease in a Charismatic evangelistic meeting.

Non-charismatic Bible groups, such as Baptists, etc., do not accept "healing" services as valid. They follow the guidelines for healing found in the New Testament book of James, which states:

> Is any sick among you?
> Let him call for the elders of the church;
> and let them pray over him,
> anointing him with oil
> in the name of the Lord:
>
> And the prayer of faith
> shall save the sick,
> and the Lord shall raise him up . . .

(James 5:14, 15)

For more on unorthodox methods of healing, read the special feature pages in this book on *How To Laugh Your Way Back To Better Health* and *Visualization Therapy.*

2

CANCER . . . SOME OF ITS CAUSES

What are some of the contemporary living areas believed to cause Cancer? Let's take them in alphabetical order.

Asbestos

We Breathe It!

Motion picture star Steve McQueen was a victim of Cancer believed caused by asbestos. How frightening to realize that the air of city streets is loaded with asbestos. The average car wears out 3 or 4 sets of asbestos brake linings and 1 or 2 asbestos clutch facings in its lifetime. Floor tiles, roofing materials, insulation board, water pipes are part of virtually thousands of products made with asbestos. It is practically indestructible. And we breathe it!

Talcum and baby powders (related to asbestos) as well as some of the feminine hygiene sprays may also cause Cancer. Dr. Keith Griffiths reported in the March, 1971 *Journal of Obstetrics and Gynecology* (British) that particles of talc were found in approximately 75% of the ovarian tumors and 50% of the cervical tumors examined.

**We
Swallow
It!**

Birth Control Pills

Dr. Otto Sartorius, Director of Cancer Control Clinic at Santa Barbara General Hospital in California reports that:

> Women who use the Pill
> are sustaining irreversible and permanent breast changes.
>
> The cancer-risk factor
> in women taking the Pill
> is 2.8 times greater
> than in women who do not use the Pill.

The synthetic chemical hormones in the Pill are given the names of female hormones, estrogen and progesterone. Research has now shown that the Pill is a proven and accepted causitive agent in Heart Disease, Diabetes and Cancer.

Women who take the Pill develop clotting diseases 4-11 times as often as women who do not.

**We
Use
It!**

Cosmetics

Many of the coloring dyes used in soaps, lipsticks and other cosmetics are considered cancer-causitive. They include: Red Nos. 2, 4, 10, 11, 12 and 13, Yellow No. 1 and Blue No. 6. Many more dyes are in question!

**We
Eat
It!**

DES (Diethylstilbestrol)

Since 1950 DES has been used as a growth stimulant in animal feeds. DES is a synthetic preparation possessing estrongenic properties. It is cancer-causitive.

Estrogen

DES has not only been used in animal feed but also prescribed for humans as a treatment of menopausal disturbances and other disorders due to estrogen deficiencies. *The New England Journal of Medicine*, December 4, 1975 reported in two independent studies that women on estrogen are from 5 to 14 times more likely to have Cancer of the uterus.

There are many medical research reports available that indicate estrogen therapy is linked to Cancer in both men and women.

Eating Habits

Cancer Caused By Some Diets

Processed foods which are loaded with food additives such as nitrites, monosodiumglutimate and other chemicals contribute to Cancer ... as does alcohol and tobacco.

Dr. Lon O. Crosby, a nutritionist with Enviro Control Inc. in Bethesda, Maryland reported that:

> *Some 40% of men's cancers
> and 60% of women's
> are estimated to be caused by diet.*
>
> *We predict that 700,000 lives
> could be saved in the year 2000
> if a nutrition program were
> implemented now.*[1]

He went on to say that a person who eats two 12-oz. charcoal-broiled steaks in a week gets more tar than from smoking

---

[1]*Medical World News*, October, 1977, p. 82.

two packs of cigarettes a day for that period.

Many cancer researchers point to a link between a high-fat diet and Cancer.

Hair Dyes

The
Price
Of
Beauty

Studies have shown that 150 of 169 permanent hair dyes tested could damage genes and, therefore, might be able to cause Cancer or birth defects. These studies were begun by Dr. Roy Shore of New York University and reported by the *Journal of National Cancer Institute.*

Fluorescent Lights

The
Penalty
Of
Progress

Scientists from the National Cancer Institute have made the unsettling discovery that the light from ordinary fluorescent lamps can cause mutations in the chromosomes of hamster cells. Some believe that this type of lighting may also affect humans transferring normal cells into cancerous ones.

Mothers' Milk

How
Tragic!

A study shows suspected Cancer-causing chemicals called PCB's have so infiltrated the nation's food supply they show in the milk of practically all mothers who breast-feed their babies. **PCB** is short for *polychlorinated biphenyls*. These are chemicals used by industry in the manufacture of paints, dyes, plastics and electrical insulation. PCB is suspected of causing Cancer in human beings even at low levels of exposure.

**Problems
Of
Environment**

Pollutants

Of the 365,000 Cancer cases reported in 1975, the majority of them could be traced to environmental sources.

New Jersey which is highly industrialized is also known for having the highest rate of Cancer in the United States. In fact, wherever there are heavy concentrations of petroleum refineries, there is a high incidence of Cancer.

Even jet planes, which burn ozone, have been targeted as a causitive-agent in Cancer. Much of the skin Cancers are linked to this. Depletion of our ozone layer shield is considered a serious threat.

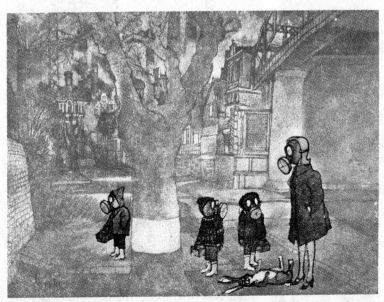

This German cartoon, although humorous, may reflect what life will be like in the year 2000.

In Tokyo, oxygen vending machines have already
been installed in coffee shops and arcades.
Dispense a whiff for 25¢.

New York City at noon. Pollutants poison the air.

Tobacco

**Lives
Lost
To**

The battle against lung cancer is being lost. During the last 25 years, death rates from this type of Cancer went up 200%. The major cause of lung cancer is cigarette smoking. And almost 1 out of every 4 Americans smokes! Not only is it hazardous to them . . . but it is hazardous to those around them who inhale the smoke as unwilling participants!

Valium

**Tranquil
Death**

The most widely prescribed drug in the world, Valium, may promote the growth of existing Cancers. Dr. David F. Horrobin in a January, 1981 meeting of the American Association for the Advancement of Science finds that *diazepam* (the chemical name for Valium)

> . . . *had actions similar to those
> of cancer promoters.*

Cancer promoters are agents that do not cause Cancer by themselves but make the body much more sensitive to other Cancer-causing agents. It is estimated that 42% of American women have taken tranquilizers of the diazepam type!

Water

**We
Drink
It!**

Because we as a society demand many material possessions, industry works overtime to spew out more and more gadgets. They then dump the left over pollutants from the manufacturing process into our lakes and rivers. Eventually,

Poor Quality Water Linked To Cancer

these chemical pollutants find their way into our body . . . sometimes through drinking water or even through mothers' milk. The University of Pennsylvania in tests on water have concluded that poor water quality is linked to stomach, colon, rectal and urinary tract Cancers.

Fluoridated water . . . the use of which is a highly controversial subject . . . is believed by many to cause Cancer.

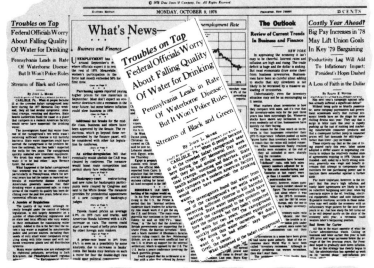

3

WHAT IS CANCER?

TIME TO STRESS PREVENTATIVES

Seeking Preventatives

After reading these brief descriptions of some things that can cause Cancer . . . you may ask yourself the question: "*Well, what doesn't cause Cancer?*"

At least this brief listing will give you some idea of the complexity of the subject. And as our society becomes more populated and industrialized and our foods become more processed . . . Cancer and other catastrophic diseases will increase.

Would it be fair to say then, that the orthodox approach will continue to be seeking to approach the problem <u>after</u> one already has Cancer? I believe so . . . but I hope not.

Would it not also be fair to say that the <u>one possible insurance</u> for cancer <u>preventative</u> would be to live in a <u>healthy</u> environment while fortifying oneself with healthy nutrients through a sound diet? I think so.

Who Can Define Cancer?

Just exactly what is Cancer?

From orthodox medicine's viewpoint, Cancer can be defined as:

A malignant tumor;
abnormal and uncontrolled
  cellular growth,
characterized by
invasion of surrounding healthy tissue
and
metastatic spread[1] to distant organs,
leading to the formation of
secondary growths

Thus modern medicine believes that Cancer is a disorderly growth of tissue cells.

Others ask: "*While it may be true that the end result producing Cancer is a disorderly growth of tissue cells . . . what actually triggers this disorderly growth?*

One nutritionist, who has been called a "quack" by the medical profession, nevertheless, says:

Cancer is premature aging
due to a mineral deficiency
in our diet!

Cancer is not like an animal
preying upon you at all!
Cancer does not actually grow as such.

As the minerals become more deficient
in your system,
your body has less resistance
and as the resistance decreases
the size of the cancer increases.

---

[1]*Metastic spread* refers to movement of cancer cells from one part of the body to another. Someone with cancer of the breast or lung, as an example, may eventually die of Cancer of the liver!

4

THE MEDICAL APPROACH TO CANCER

**Three
Orthodox
Approaches**

There are _three_ major orthodox treatments for Cancer: Chemotherapy, Surgery and Radiotherapy _(also known as Cobalt therapy)_.

Chemotherapy (1)

Chemotherapy is frequently used along with x-ray radiation or with hormone therapy. Chemotherapy literally means _treatment with chemicals._ There are many types of chemicals used. They are given either orally, by injection into a muscle or subcutaneous tissue, or by intravenous infusion. Most of these drugs can be given in your doctor's office or at a hospital's out-patient department.

The length of chemotherapy treatment varies from several months to 2 years, depending on your response to the drug. You may tolerate chemotherapy better if you eat a light meal before and after the procedure.

As to the value of chemotherapy there are many opinions. Chemotherapy has had a

CANCER DEATHS ESTIMATED YEARLY BY TYPE AND SEX

Male:
- Skin 2%
- Oral 3%
- Lung 34%
- Colon & Rectum 12%
- Pancreas 5%
- Prostate 10%
- Urinary 5%
- Leukemia & Lymphomas 9%
- All other 20%

Female:
- Skin 1%
- Oral 1%
- Breast 19%
- Lung 15%
- Colon & Rectum 15%
- Pancreas 5%
- Ovary 6%
- Uterus 5%
- Urinary 3%
- All other 21%
- Leukemia & Lymphomas 9%

measure of success in treatment of some blood malignancies such as leukemia and Hodgkin's disease.

Robert E. Rothenberg, M.D., F.A.C.S. says:

> There is an every-increasing number of chemicals and drugs that have been found effective in slowing down the growth of Cancers and allied conditions. Although these chemicals rarely can produce complete and permanent destruction of the malignancy, they frequently are successful in prolonging life.[1]

Side Effects Abound

Many drugs prescribed to battle Cancer cause numerous side effects and even death. One, _cyclophosphamide_ (Cytoxan, Procytox), actually causes Cancer. The cancer drug _doxorubicin hydrochloride_ (Adriamycin) causes heart damage that could prove fatal.

> The goal of chemotherapy is to destroy every Cancer cell in the patient's body by interfering with neoplastic cell division (abnormal cell division). However, each dose of an antineoplastic drug destroys only a fraction of neoplastic cells, since only a fraction of the cells are dividing when the drug is given. Therefore treatment must be given very early and be prolonged. The doses needed to obtain maximum therapeutic response are quite toxic.[2]

[1]Robert E. Rothenberg, The Complete Surgical Guide, (New York: Weathervane Books), 1974, pp. 220, 221.

[2]Nurse's Guide To Drugs, (Horsham, Pennsylvania: Intermed Communications, Inc.), 1980, p. 748.

BE AWARE OF SIDE EFFECTS

**Complications
May Follow**

The Medical Letter, a non-profit publication on Drugs and Therapeutics issued primarily to physicians reports:

> The complications of chemotherapy frequently include severe nausea and vomiting and infections and hemorrhage due to bone marrow depression.
>
> In addition, hyperuricemia[1] can occur due to treatment-induced destruction of large numbers of tumor cells, although allopurinol can usually prevent this complication.
>
> Also, many anticancer drugs may themselves be carcinogenic (SM Sieber et al., Adv. Cancer Res., 22:57, 1975).
> Virtually all of the drugs used in cancer chemotherapy are potentially harmful to the fetus if taken during pregnancy; women of childbearing age should be warned to avoid conception while they are being treated with these agents.[2]

**Adverse
Reactions**

The chemical agents in chemotherapy can destroy huge numbers of white blood cells and interfere with the body's natural defense mechanism. In some cases, the use

---

[1]Hyperuricemia is an abnormal amount of uric acid in the blood.

[2]The Medical Letter (New Rochelle, New York: The Medical Letter, Inc.), September 22, 1978, pp. 81, 82.

of chemotherapy may trigger an over-whelming infection and the patient may die sooner than without such therapy.

NAUSEA

Loss Of Appetite

Nausea, vomiting and loss of appetite (*anorexia*) are the most common side effects of chemotherapy treatment. Sometimes severe nausea and vomiting can continue for days without relief, *The Medical Letter* reports. They also state:

> Delta-9-tetrahydrocannabinol (THC), the main active ingredient of marihuana can relieve these symptoms in some patients who do not respond to other antiemetic drugs. The adverse effects include drowsiness, which can be disabling. Some patients complain of dry mouth, dizziness, inability to concentrate or disorientation.[1]

Antiemetics (antinauseants) to prevent nausea, include such drugs as Antivert, Benadryl, Compazine, Donnatal, Librax and Tigan. Side effects vary with each of these drugs from drowsiness, dry mouth, fainting, absence of menstruation, skin disorders, constipation, changes in sex drive to difficulty in urination.

Patients are advised to eat well even if they do not have an appetite. A nutritious diet lessens toxicity and speeds recovery from adverse reactions of drugs.

[1]The Medical Letter (New Rochelle, New York: The Medical Letter, Inc.), May 16, 1980, pp. 41, 42.

Oral Side Effects include dry mouth with ulcers. Medicated rinses are used with Lidocaine viscous, an oral anesthetic rinse.

HAIR AND SKIN DAMAGE

Scalp
Hypothermia
To Avoid
Hair Loss

Hair and skin damage are common side effects. Alopecia (partial or complete loss of hair) can be distressing to a patient. It is possible to lose some or all of his hair . . . not only scalp hair, but eyelashes, eyebrows, underarm and pubic hair. The hair, however, should grow back about 8 weeks after therapy has stopped.

At some hospitals *"scalp hypothermia"* treatments are used to eliminate or minimize hair loss. The treatment involves filling an ordinary plastic bag with crushed ice and keeping it in place around a patient's head with a turban of bandages for 35 minutes. It is put on five minutes before an injection of doxorubicin (Adriamycin, Adria) and kept on for another 30 minutes when the drug is considered most active. In their research, one group noted that normally 95% of their patients lose their hair during chemotherapy treatments. But with the cold-scalp treatments (on 13 people), eight patients lost less than 25% of their hair and four lost 25% to 50%. Three got moderate protection and two received no benefit.[1]

[1]Cool-headed Cancer Patients Keep Hair, *Medical World News*, May 14, 1979, p. 19.

5

DRUGS USED IN CHEMOTHERAPY

**5
Basic
Drugs**

There are **5** basic drug categories used in chemotherapy treatments. Each category has a specific use. **All have side effects.**

1. Alkylating agents

**Developed
From
Mustard Gas**

It may surprise you to learn this family of Cancer drugs was developed from the military research done on mustard gas!

Mechlorethamine hydrochloride (nitrogen mustard) is used sometimes for treatment of lymphomas and some leukemias and sacormas. Alkylating agents can act during any phase of a cell's life cycle which gives them an advantage over other drugs. An alkylating agent is one that introduces an alkyl radical into a compound in place of a hydrogen atom. They attack the DNA by either binding or breaking the chains apart.

Side effects may include hair loss, gastrointestinal irritation, hemorrhagic cystitis and possible bone marrow depression.

2. Antimetabolites

Not Intelligent

These drugs are antitumor agents. They are designed to block cell division. The aim is to prevent cells, including Cancer cells from reproducing and surviving.

Antimetabolites are not intelligent drugs. They destroy healthy as well as diseased cells.

Side effects may include gastric and oral ulcers, anemia, bone marrow depression, nausea.

3. Antibiotic antineoplastic agents

Possible Depression

These drugs are designed to stop Cancer cell production by interrupting protein synthesis.

Side effects may include loss of appetite, anemia, skin redness or eruptions, hair loss, depression and possibly pneumonitis.

4. Antineoplastics altering hormone balance

Affects Sex Drive

These drugs either repress or stimulate changes in the hormonal balance of the body.

Side effects for women may include clitoral enlargement, increased sex drive, hair loss, nausea and acne.

5. Vinca alkaloids and asparaginase

**For
Breast
Cancer**

The elements used to make this drug are taken from the periwinkle plant. Its treatment comes from folklore. It is thought to arrest cell division. Asparaginase is given intravenously or intramuscularly. It is used frequently for breast or testicular cancer.

Side effects may include nausea, depression, fatigue, confusion, weight loss, rash, ulcers, constipation and phlebitis.

Perhaps after reading the possible side effects of these drugs you may wonder at the value of chemotherapy. We have listed only a few of the side effects in each category. There are many others.

Understanding CHEMOTHERAPY DRUGS

Any drug effect other than what is therapeutically intended can be called a side effect. It may be expected and benign, or unexpected and potentially harmful. . . . A side effect may be tolerated for a necessary therapeutic effect or it may be hazardous and unacceptable, and require discontinuation of the drug. . . . Most important, patients need to be told what side effects to expect so they won't become worried or even stop taking the drug on their own.

Nurse's Guide To Drugs/page 19
Intermed Communications, Inc.

NAME	Possible SIDE EFFECTS	Other CONSIDERATIONS
Alkylating agents		
busulfan Myleran	Anemia, nausea, vomiting, diarrhea, testicular atrophy, impotence, loss of hair, enlargement of male breasts.	Side effects may be delayed for 6 months. Persistent cough may develop.
carmustine (BCNU) BiCNU	Cumulative bone marrow depression, nausea (can be severe), intense pain at injection site, kidney disease, lung inflammation.	Fever, sore throat, fatigue, and anemia may appear. Should not be mixed with other drugs during administration. Avoid contact with skin.
chlorambucil Leukeran	Abnormal decrease of white blood corpuscles, anemia, may cause sterility, excessive amounts of potassium in blood, scaling of skin tissue, nausea.	Should not be given for at least 4 weeks after radiation or other chemotherapy. Best administered before breakfast or at bedtime to reduce nausea.
cis-platinum Platinol	Inflammation of surface nerves, loss of taste, seizures, hearing loss, nausea, vomiting, abnormal amount of uric acid in the blood.	Report hearing loss immediately to prevent permanent hearing loss. A hearing test should be given before and during treatment. Nausea and vomiting may be severe for 24 hours.
cylophosphamide Cytoxan Procytox	Abnormal decrease of white blood corpuscles, anemia, loss of appetite, nausea and vomiting, inflammation of the mouth, inability of ovaries or male sex glands or testes to function, hemorrhagic cystitis, sterility, hair loss, hepatitis.	Avoid getting pregnant. Drug can affect fetus. Use contraceptives while taking this drug and for 4 months thereafter. Cystitis can occur months after therapy has stopped.
dacarbazine DTIC-Dome	Severe nausea, excessive amount of potassium in blood, loss of appetite, metallic taste in mouth, flu-like symptoms may last 7-21 days, swelling (in children), hair loss, facial flushing.	Don't give food 2-6 hours before giving drug. Watch for signs of bleeding.

NAME	Possible SIDE EFFECTS	Other CONSIDERATIONS
lomustine (CCNU) CeeNU	Abnormal decrease of white blood corpuscles, anemia, lethargy, lack of coordination, nausea, vomiting, excessive amount of potassium in blood, hair loss.	Nausea may last 24 hours. Should be given at least 6 weeks apart. Watch closely for signs of bleeding.
mechlorethamine hydrochloride Mustargen	Abnormal decrease in number of blood platelets, temporary speech difficulties, possible slurred speech, convulsions, progressive muscular paralysis, ringing in the ears, metallic taste in mouth, possible deafness in high doses, nausea, vomiting, loss of appetite, blood clots in the veins (thrombophlebitis), hair loss.	Avoid drug contact with skin. Drug is very unstable and should be prepared for use within 15 minutes. May cause an acute infectious disease of the spinal nerves called *Herpes Zoster.*
melphalan Alkeran	Abnormal decrease in number of blood platelets, abnormal decrease in white blood corpuscles, anemia, high fever, possible ulcers in mouth, rectum and vagina, loss of appetite, nausea, vomiting.	Excellent mouth care should be given.
pipobroman Vercyte	Abnormal decrease in white blood corpuscles, abnormal decrease in number of blood platelets, anemia, nausea, vomiting, cramping, diarrhea, loss of appetite, skin rash.	May destroy red blood cells.
thiotepa Thiotepa	Abnormal decrease of white blood corpuscles, abnormal decrease in number of blood platelets, anemia, abnormally small number of neutrophil cells in the blood, deficiency of lymphocytes in the blood, nausea, vomiting, loss of appetite, absence or suppression of menstruation, intense pain at injection site, hives, rash, headache, fever, dizziness.	May require use of local anesthetic at injection site. Toxic effects may be delayed or prolonged.
uracil mustard	Bone marrow depression, abnormal decrease in number of blood platelets, abnormal decrease of white blood corpuscles, anemia, mental confusion, irritability, nervousness and depression, nausea, vomiting, diarrhea, loss of appetite, absence or suppression of menstruation, hair loss, severe itching, skin rash.	Usually given at bedtime to reduce nausea. Watch for signs of skin hemorrhage.

Antimetabolites

NAME	Possible SIDE EFFECTS	Other CONSIDERATIONS
azathioprine Imuran	Abnormal decrease of white blood corpuscles, bone marrow depression, anemia, abnormal decrease in number of blood platelets, retina disorders, nausea, vomiting, loss of appetite, inflammation of pancreas, mouth ulcers, inflammation of esophagus, skin rash, joint pains, hair loss, hepatitis, jaundice.	Be alert for clay-colored stools, dark urine, yellow skin. Report any mild infections such as sore throat, fever or fatigue. Avoid conception up to 4 months after stopping treatment.
cytarbine (ARA-C, cytosine arabinoside) Cytosar	Abnormal decrease of white blood corpuscles, anemia, nausea, vomiting, diarrhea, ulcers in mouth, difficulty in swallowing, phlebitis, possible blood poisoning.	Requires excellent mouth care to minimize side effects in oral area.

NAME	Possible SIDE EFFECTS	Other CONSIDERATIONS
floxuridine FUDR	Abnormal decrease of white blood corpuscles, anemia, abnormal decrease in number of blood platelets, mental confusion, difficulty in maintaining equilibrium (vertigo), convulsions, depression, hiccups, fatigue, constant involuntary cyclical movement of the eyeball, possible paralysis of one half of the body, blurred vision, nausea, cramps, vomiting, diarrhea, bleeding, duodenal ulcer, skin rash, possible blood poisoning.	Should not be given to one in poor nutrition state. Should be discontinued if there are severe skin reactions or distress in the gastro-intestinal area.
fluorouracil **(5-fluorouracil)** Adrucil, 5-FU	Abnormal decrease of white blood corpuscles, abnormal decrease in number of blood platelets, anemia, angina, blurred vision and eye irritation, inflammation of eyes with unusual intolerance to light, inflammation of the mouth, nausea, vomiting, diarrhea, skin rash, changes in nails, weakness, hair loss.	Report any inflammation of the mouth or diarrhea. May indicate dosage too strong. Eyes should be protected by glasses that block sun's strong rays. Report any chest pain.
hydroxyurea Hydrea	Abnormal decrease of white blood corpuscles, abnormal decrease in number of blood platelets, bone marrow depression, drowsiness, loss of appetite, nausea, vomiting, diarrhea, inflammation of the mouth, skin rash, severe itching.	May cause hearing and visual hallucinations.
mercapto- **purine** Purinethol	Abnormal decrease of white blood corpuscles, abnormal decrease in number of blood platelets, nausea, vomiting, loss of appetite, painful mouth ulcers, diminished amount of urine flow, abnormal amount of uric acid in the blood, rash, jaundice.	Drug should be discontinued if there is nausea and vomiting because of toxicity.
methotrexate **sodium** Mexate	Abnormal decrease of white blood corpuscles, abnormal decrease in number of blood platelets, anemia, destruction of the myelin sheath of nerve tissue in the brain area may occur a few years later, inflammation of the mouth, diarrhea leading possibly to intestinal perforation, psoriatic lesions, hair loss and possible chromosome damage.	Avoid conception during or immediately following treatment. Mouth ulcers or other side effects may require stopping drug. Patient should be weighed weekly. Avoid sun exposure without proper sun glasses.
thioguanine Lanvis	Abnormal decrease of white blood corpuscles, abnormal decrease in number of blood platelets, anemia, nausea, vomiting, inflammation of the mouth, diarrhea, loss of appetite, jaundice.	Drug should be stopped if liver tenderness occurs or signs of jaundice.

NAME	Possible SIDE EFFECTS	Other CONSIDERATIONS

Antibiotic antineoplastic agents

NAME	Possible SIDE EFFECTS	Other CONSIDERATIONS
bleomycin sulfate Blenoxane	Abnormal decrease of white blood corpuscles, abnormal decrease in number of blood platelets, abnormal sensitivity of scalp and fingers, headache, inflammation of the mouth, loss of appetite, nausea, vomiting, diarrhea, shedding of skin on hands, feet and pressure areas, loss of hair, swelling of joints, fever, cough, chills, below normal blood pressure.	Vitamin C may aid skin side effects. Report any inflammation in lung area immediately.
dactinomycin (actinomycin D) Cosmegen	Abnormal decrease of white blood corpuscles, abnormal decrease in number of blood platelets, anemia, loss of appetite, nausea, vomiting, abdominal pain, diarrhea, inflammation of the mouth, inflammation of the lip, inflammation of the tongue, inflammation of the rectum and anus, phlebitis, severe damage to soft tissue, shedding of skin, acne-like eruptions, loss of hair, fatigue, muscle pains.	Report inflammation of mouth, diarrhea immediately. May require stopping treatment.
doxorubicin hydrochloride Adriamycin	Abnormal decrease of white blood corpuscles, abnormal decrease in number of blood platelets, congestive heart failure, irregular heart beat, nausea, vomiting, diarrhea, inflammation of the mouth and esophagus, red-colored urine, complete hair loss within 3 to 4 weeks. Hair may regrow 2-5 months after drug is stopped.	Warn patient that inflammation of the esophagus is common and that hair loss will occur.
mithramycin Mithracin	Abnormal decrease in number of blood platelets, bleeding, drowsiness, irritability, dizziness, headache, facial flushing, depression, nausea, vomiting, loss of appetite, diarrhea, inflammation of the mouth, eye inflammation, skin irritation, fatigue, fever.	Report signs of bleeding.
mitomycin Mutamycin	Abnormal decrease in number of blood platelets, abnormal decrease of white blood corpuscles, hemorrhage, numbness, prickling and tingling sensations, nausea, vomiting, loss of appetite, inflammation of the mouth, kidney failure may occur several months later, shedding of skin, loss of hair, fever, cough, difficulty in breathing.	Can cause serious lung problems.

NAME	Possible SIDE EFFECTS	Other CONSIDERATIONS
procarbazine hydrochloride Matulane Natulan	Abnormal decrease of white blood corpuscles, anemia, headache, dizziness, nervousness, depression, insomnia, nightmares, confusion, convulsions, hallucinations, coma, lack of muscle coordination, abnormal touch sensations, tremors, weakness, hoarseness, nausea, vomiting, loss of appetite, inflammation of the mouth, diarrhea, constipation, difficulty in swallowing, skin rash, loss of hair, jaundice, excessive sweating, cough.	At least one month should elapse after radiation or other chemotherapy before starting treatment of this drug.
Antineoplastics altering hormone balance		
calusterone Methosarb	Clitoral enlargement, nausea, vomiting, excessive amount of calcium in the blood, acne, oily skin, facial hair, development of male characteristics, possible increased sex drive, hair loss, jaundice, fever.	Temperature should be taken daily. Inadvisable for premenopausal women unless ovaries no longer functioning.
dromostano-lene propionate Drolban	Clitoral enlargement, excessive amount of calcium in the blood, acne, deepened voice, facial hair growth, development of male characteristics, possible increased sex drive, pain at injection site.	Results of this drug are not immediate and may be delayed 8-12 weeks. Should not be used in male breast cancer nor in premenopausal women.
mitotane Lysodren	Prolonged sleepiness, depression, difficulty in maintaining equilibrium (vertigo), possible brain damage, severe nausea, vomiting diarrhea, loss of appetite, skin rash.	Drug should be stopped if it causes shock or injury. Those who are overweight experience longer-lasting side effects.
tamoxifen citrate Nolvadex	Nausea, vomiting, loss of appetite, vaginal discharge and bleeding, skin rash, appearance of breast milk, hot flashes.	Should be used cautiously where there is an abnormal decrease in number of blood platelets or white blood corpuscles.
Vinca alkaloids and asparaginase		
asparaginase Elspar	Abnormal decrease of white blood corpuscles, abnormal decrease in number of blood platelets, sleepiness, depression, coma, confusion, irritability, headaches, hallucinations, vomiting which may last up to 24 hours, loss of appetite, nausea, cramps, loss of weight, increased blood urea, possible kidney failure, abnormal amount of sugar in urine, increased urination, skin rash, hives, fever.	Must be administered in hospital with professional supervision. Advise if fever arises or bleeding occurs.

NAME	Possible SIDE EFFECTS	Other CONSIDERATIONS
vinblastine sulfate (VLB) Velban	Abnormal decrease of white blood corpuscles, abnormal decrease in number of blood platelets, severe drop in white blood cell count, depression, numbness, prickling and tingling sensations, neuritis, muscle pain and weakness, dizziness, convulsions, headache, abnormal rapidity of heart beat, inflammation of pharynx, nausea, vomiting, inflammation of mouth, ulcer and bleeding, constipation and diarrhea, loss of appetite, loss of weight, abdominal pains, deficient amount of sperm in seminal fluid, inability to ejaculate semen, urinary retention, phlebitis, possibility of hair loss, low fever, light sensitivity.	Report immediately if mouth inflammation occurs. Should not be given closer than 7 days apart! Caution: Do not confuse vinblastine with vincristine!
vincristine sulfate Oncovin	Anemia, abnormal decrease of white blood corpuscles, abnormal decrease in number of blood platelets, sensory loss, numbness, prickling and tingling sensations, wrist and foot drop, inability to coordinate muscles, headache, jaw pain, hoarseness with possible vocal cord paralysis, visual disturbances, muscle weakness, depression, cramps, insomnia, coma, convulsions, hallucinations, high blood pressure, constipation, nausea, vomiting, loss of appetite, inflammation of mouth, loss of weight, difficulty in swallowing, increased urination, painful or difficult urination, phlebitis, loss of hair.	Should not be given closer than 7 days apart! Stool softener and laxative often recommended.

For complete listing of side effects and contraindications, medical professionals should refer to:

Physicians' Desk Reference (PDR)
Medical Economics Company
Oradell, New Jersey, 07649

Nurse's Guide To Drugs
Intermed Communications, Inc.
1111 Bethlehem Pike
Springhouse, Pennsylvania 19477

Both of these books are revised annually and new updated editions are available each year.

6

CANCER AND SURGERY

SURGERY Used in Cancer ②

**Surgery
Can Be
Extensive**

Cancer surgery usually involves not only the excision of the diseased organ but also removal of the connective tissues, lymph channels and lymph nodes that drain the cancerous site.

All qualified surgeons are trained to do Cancer surgery.

A physician can not always tell whether a tumor is benign *(not malignant or recurrent)* or malignant when he removes it in surgery. That is why a small part of the tumor tissue is taken for study. Two methods are available: quick-frozen biopsy and microscopic biopsy.

**Biopsy
Required**

A **quick-frozen biopsy** is one where the tissue involved is quick-frozen in order to make it suitable for immediate microscopic examination. This can be done even while the patient is in the operating room ... as the answer to whether the tumor is benign or malignant only takes 15-20 minutes. Frozen or quick-frozen section biopsy is not always accurate.

A **needle biopsy** is not as accurate as a quick-frozen biopsy where tissue is examined. The reason: the amount of tissue that can be obtained from needle withdrawal is sometimes so small that it makes interpretation difficult.

A regular microscopic biopsy done at a laboratory usually takes from 3 to 7 days.

**Time
Is Only
Assurance**

The most accepted way of telling whether surgery has resulted in a permanent cure is by the passage of time. Few Cancers recur after a 5-10 year period.

The size of the tumor does not indicate that it is benign of malignant. A very large tumor can be perfectly benign. Nor can a surgeon know for sure, in many instances, whether he has totally removed the cancerous growth. That is why Cancer surgery is more extensive. The trend today is to seek to resolve Cancer not by surgery but, preferably by hormone or chemotherapy treatment.

7

DOES THE MEDICAL APPROACH
DESTROY NUTRITION CHANNELS?

**Too
Late
For
Nutrition?**

Some nutritionists believe that once a chemotherapy program is completed by a patient . . . a nutritional therapy program will be ineffective. They believe that chemotherapy destroys the nutrient-carrying vessels of the body. Thus your body is unable to absorb the valuable minerals, vitamins and other nutrients needed to combat the condition which caused the Cancer.

**Rate Of
Cancer
Increasing**

Proponents of orthodox medicine do not accept a nutrition program as a valid primary therapy for the treatment of Cancer. They rely instead on chemotherapy, surgery and cobalt therapy as prime approaches to the problem.

The problem is that more people are dying of Cancer in every age group than at any other time in our history. In two years alone, lung cancer increased 13%; breast cancer increased 17%; stomach cancer increased 28% and prostate cancer increased 32%. These figures are findings of the National Cancer Institute!

COBALT THERAPY ③

**Can
Affect
Normal
Tissue**

Cobalt is a part of Vitamin B_{12} and a deficiency of cobalt leads to anemia.

Radioactive cobalt therapy has supplanted the conventional x-ray therapy in most hospitals. The reason: cobalt radiation has greater penetrating power and causes less damage to skin and tissues.

Cobalt therapy is not painful but there may be some temporary side effects. When radiation is applied to a tumor or other abnormal cell it makes those cells unable to function normally. Cobalt is generally used after surgery to make sure cancer cells are destroyed.

Normal tissue is also affected by the cobalt treatment but while tumor tissue dies, normal tissue generally recovers.

HYPERTHERMIA

**Healing
By Heat**

Thermotherapy . . . the killing of tumors with heat . . . offers some hope when all else has failed.

Heat makes certain cancers more operable, more radiosensitive and more susceptible to drugs.

Thermotherapy and Hyperthermia, in particular, is based on the supposition that as temperatures go up, cancer cells die sooner than healthy ones. This belief is controversial. Hyperthermia then is *the*

HYPERTHERMIA CENTERS

Hyperthermia therapy is only done at a limited number of health centers in the United States.

Middle Atlantic
Memorial Sloan-Kettering Cancer Center
New York City

Roswell Park Memorial Institute
Buffalo, New York

South
National Cancer Institute
Bethesda, Maryland

University of Mississippi School of Medicine
Jackson, Mississippi

Midwest
Indiana University School of Medicine
Indianapolis, Indiana

Southwest
University of Arizona Health Sciences Center
Tucson, Arizona

University of New Mexico School of Medicine
Albuquerque, New Mexico

St. Joseph Hospital
Houston, Texas

Pacific
University of California School of Medicine
Los Angeles, California

Stanford University Hospital
Stanford, California

Hyperthermia is considered by some a last resort treatment. The risk of death from this treatment is close to 10% when whole-body heating is employed.

treatment of disease by raising body temperature.

Promising Results

Two hyperthermia patients treated at the University of Arizona showed promising results from this approach. One, a 54-year-old housewife who had a radical mastectomy in 1968 developed surface nodules after 6 years. Chemotherapy, x-ray therapy and surgery were ineffective. Hyperthermia treatments had significant healing effect on the nodules.

A 34-year-old woman with a painful, bleeding vaginal cancer was treated by hyperthermia. The tumor dwindled to 10% of its original size. These reports were made in Medical World News, May 14, 1979, pp. 52-69.

INTERFERON

Not Really A Miracle Drug?

There are more than a million Cancer patients in the United States and 600,000 new ones are added each year. Is it any wonder that the hint of a miracle cure brings instant and impassioned inquiries from patients and their families.

As medical reporter, Alice Barrus reports:

> *Great hopes are being held out for a protein produced in minuscule amounts by the human body's own cells: interferon.*
>
> *As deployed by the body, interferon is an extraordinarily potent agent. It protects (uninfected) cells against attack by viruses,*

slows the growth of cells and affects, in complex ways, the operation of the body's other natural defense mechanisms.[1]

**Results
Not
Conclusive**

The American Cancer Society has treated 102 patients using interferon for four different types of Cancer: non-Hodgkin's lymphoma, breast cancer, skin cancer and bone-marrow cancer. Twenty-five percent of the patients showed *"objective improvement."* Their tumors have regressed 50% or more. All of these cancer victims had previously failed to respond to conventional forms of treatment.

The theory is that interferon somehow prods healthy cells to produce defenses against the invasion of diseased cells.

---

[1]Alice Barruss, The Exciting Promise of Interferon, (Indianapolis, Indiana: The Saturday Evening Post), March, 1981, pp. 77-80.

8

LUNG, COLON AND PROSTATE CANCER

LUNG CANCER

**Smokers
Tempting
Death**

Those who smoke cigarettes are *ten times more prone than nonsmokers to develop lung cancer.*[1] Lung cancer develops without you having any real initial symptoms. Late symptoms include:

> *loss of appetite*
> *chest pain*
> *coughing of blood*
> *weight loss*

The main treatment for lung cancer is surgical. In surgery, either the entire lung (pneumonectomy) is removed or the entire lobe of the lung (lobectomy). Too often, however, the majority of patients reach the surgeon after the Cancer has already spread to other areas. In these cases the lung is not removed and x-ray treatment is started.

---

[1]Robert E. Rothenberg, M.D., F.A.C.S., The Complete Surgical Guide. (New York: Weathervane Books), 1974, p. 557.

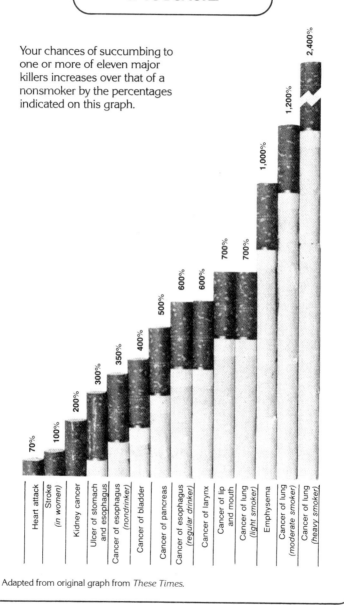

IF YOU SMOKE

Your chances of succumbing to one or more of eleven major killers increases over that of a nonsmoker by the percentages indicated on this graph.

70% Heart attack
100% Stroke *(in women)*
200% Kidney cancer
300% Ulcer of stomach and esophagus
350% Cancer of esophagus *(nondrinker)*
400% Cancer of bladder
500% Cancer of pancreas
600% Cancer of esophagus *(regular drinker)*
600% Cancer of larynx
700% Cancer of lip and mouth
700% Cancer of lung *(light smoker)*
1,000% Emphysema
1,200% Cancer of lung *(moderate smoker)*
2,400% Cancer of lung *(heavy smoker)*

Adapted from original graph from *These Times.*

COLON CANCER

**Men
More
Affected**

The colon is the large intestine ...
measures about 59 inches long and would
resemble an upright horseshoe. Two main
tumors can be present in the colon or
large intestine: *adenomas* (or *polyps*) and
the malignant growth termed a Cancer.

Some 10-15 adults have adenomas or
polyps. These can be removed without
problem and are benign. The reason they
are removed is that some have a tendency
to become cancerous.

Men have a higher incidence of bowel
cancer and it usually occurs after age 40.
Symptoms of Cancer of the bowel include:

> *anemia*
> *loss of weight and strength*
> *abdominal lump*
> *repeated bleeding from rectum*
> *change in bowel habits*
>   *with increasing constipation*

Medical treatment consists primarily in
prompt surgical removal of the affected
portion. Surgery requires advance preparation. Several days before the operation,
a low-residue diet is given and a program
of cleansing enemas.

**Less
Colostomies
Performed**

The greatest fear a patient has when he is
told he must have colon surgery is that a
colostomy may be performed. It is initially
depressing to think one will have to live
with a bowel opening on his abdominal

COLON CANCER

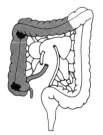

11%
Cecum and ascending colon

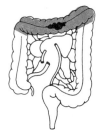

4.5%
Transverse colon

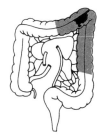

3%
Splenic flexure

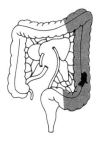

5%
Descending colon
and upper sigmoid

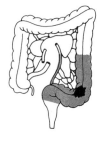

20.5%
Low sigmoid
and upper rectum

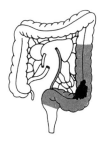

52.9%
Rectal

Chart indicates approximate incidence of cancer of the colon in each of six segments. Also shown are areas where cancer usually occurs.

wall. However, more and more operations are being performed not using the colostomy procedure . . . and in many cases, a colostomy is only a temporary measure until a second-stage operation.

PROSTATE CANCER

A Disease Of Men Over 40

The prostate gland surrounds the neck of the bladder and the uretha in the male. It is enclosed in a fibrous capsule containing smooth muscle fibers in its inner layer. The gland secretes a thin milky translucent fluid which forms part of the semen. (Semen includes sperm cells).

The majority of men, in the 40's, generally experience a benign enlargement of the prostate. As this prostate enlarges, it presses upon the urethra and obstructs the outflow of urine from the bladder. Symptoms can include:

> *increased frequency of urination*
> *need to urinate during sleeping hours*
> *decrease in the*
> *size and force*
> *of the urinary stream*
> *dribbling after completion*

If this problem becomes acute it can affect the kidneys causing kidney failure and uremia.

Can Effect Sex Drive

Cancer of the prostate occurs most often in men beyond 60 years of age. If discovered early, it can be cured. Prostate examination annually for men over 50 is recommended.

Enlargement of the prostate does not interfere with sexual relations. Surgery on the prostate can interfere with sexual potency. There are 6 different surgical operations.[1]

Hemorrhoids Do Not Turn To Cancer

Hemorrhoids (piles) <u>never</u> turn into Cancer. Benign tumor operations generally require anywhere from a day or two to a 10-12 day hospital stay. Malignant tumor operations of the colon may be done in two or three stages and may require 2-3 week stays. In a major operation, generally nothing is taken by mouth for 3 or 4 days after the operation. Bowel function returns in 4-7 days. Sexual relations can resume within 2 months.

---

[1]For complete Medical and Nutritional Approach to Prostate Problems . . . write for the book in this series titled **The Prostate.** Send $5 plus $1 for postage to Salem Kirban, Inc., Kent Road, Huntingdon Valley, Pennsylvania 19006.

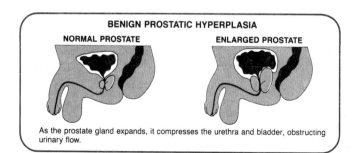

BENIGN PROSTATIC HYPERPLASIA

NORMAL PROSTATE   ENLARGED PROSTATE

As the prostate gland expands, it compresses the urethra and bladder, obstructing urinary flow.

Illustration reprinted with permission from Diseases, copyright © 1981, Intermed Communications, Inc.

How to examine your breasts

1 **In the shower:**
Examine your breasts during bath or shower; hands glide easier over wet skin. Fingers flat, move gently over every part of each breast. Use right hand to examine left breast, left hand for right breast. Check for any lump, hard knot or thickening.

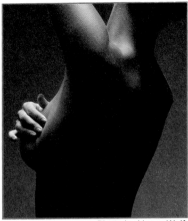

Photo by Henry Wolf

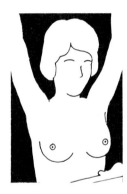

2 **Before a mirror:**
Inspect your breasts with arms at your sides. Next, raise your arms high overhead. Look for any changes in contour of each breast . . . a swelling, dimpling of skin or changes in the nipple. Then, squeeze the nipple of each breast gently between thumb and index finger. Any discharge, clear or bloody, should be reported to your doctor immediately.

3 **Lying down:**
To examine your right breast, put a pillow or folded towel under your right shoulder. Place right hand behind your head. (This distributes breast tissue more evenly on the chest. With left hand, fingers flat, press gently in small circular motions around an imaginary clock.

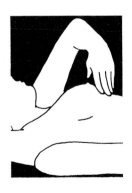

Begin at the outermost top of your right breast for 12 o'clock . . . then move to the 1 o'clock position and so on around the circle back to 12. A ridge of firm tissue in the lower curve of each breast is normal.

Then move in an inch . . . toward your nipple . . . keep circling to examine every part of your breast, including the nipple. This requires at least 3 more circles. Repeat procedure on your left breast with a pillow under your left shoulder and left hand behind head.

Courtesy American Cancer Society, Inc.

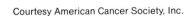

The stomach

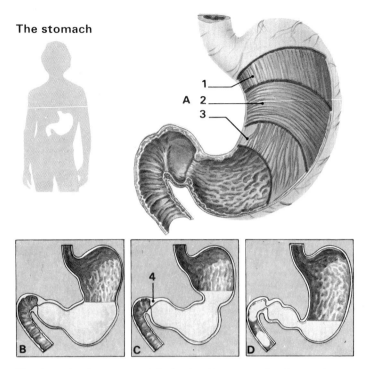

A
1
2
3

B

C
4

D

The stomach acts as a reservoir for food and has a capacity of two and a half pints. Within the stomach, solid food material is churned and kneaded for about three hours until it becomes a semiliquid mass known as chyme. The chyme is then forced into the small intestine, where the process of digestion is completed. The wall of the stomach (**A**) has three muscular layers, an outer longitudinal layer (**1**), a middle circular layer (**2**) and an inner oblique layer (**3**) As the stomach fills with food, wavelike contractions of the wall begin (**B**), and as these waves move along the stomach wall (**C**) some of the food is passed through the relaxed muscle valve at the base (**4**) and into the duodenum (**D**), the first part of the small intestine, where it is further digested before being absorbed into the body.

Mitchell Beazley Publishers, Ltd., England Atlas of the Body and Mind, Copyright © Mitchell Beazley Publishers, Ltd. 1976. Published in U.S.A. by Rand McNally & Company.

The digestive system

From the mouth, food passes down the throat into the stomach, where a churning action mixes it into a semiliquid mass.

It is then forced into the small intestine, where the major part of digestion and absorption occurs.

Undigested material passes into the large intestine, where most of the remaining water is absorbed by the bloodstream.

Solid waste collects in the rectum and is expelled through the anus.

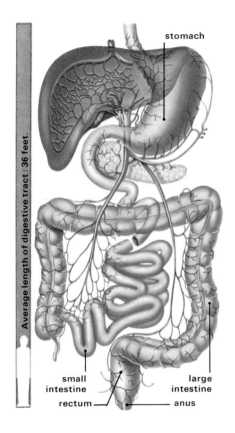

Average length of digestive tract: 36 feet.

stomach

small intestine

rectum

large intestine

anus

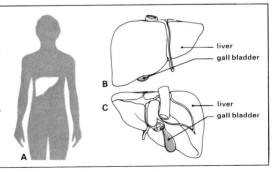

The liver and gall bladder are positioned close to each other high up in the abdomen (**A**). In the front view (**B**), the gall bladder cannot be clearly seen as it lies tucked underneath the liver. In the back view of the liver (**C**), however, the pear-shaped gall bladder is clearly visible. The liver produces bile juice, which passes down the hepatic duct to be stored in the gall bladder. Periodically, bile is released into the duodenum, where it aids the digestion of fats and neutralizes the acidity of chyme—food partly digested in the stomach.

liver

gall bladder

B

C

liver

gall bladder

A

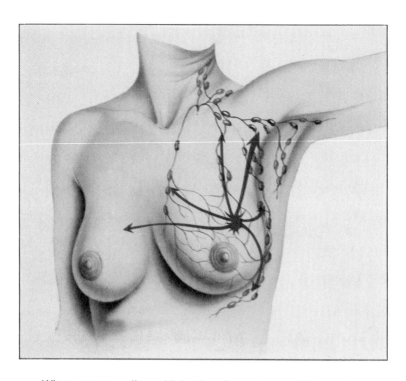

When cancer cells multiply, they form a lump. If it is not removed, the cancer may spread through the lymphatic system, a network of channels that carry fluid to the lymph nodes, where it is filtered. If malignant cells are found in these nodes—some of which are clustered around the breast, under the breastbone, above the collarbone, and in the armpit—the nodes are removed.

Opposite page . . . various kinds of surgery for breast cancer. Black lines indicate incisions.

1. Removal of the tumor and part of surrounding healthy tissue.
2. Removal of the quarter of the breast containing the tumor, plus armpit lymph nodes and some chest muscle.
3. Removal of the breast, the nodes, and some chest muscle.
4. Removal of the breast, lymph nodes, and all underlying muscle.

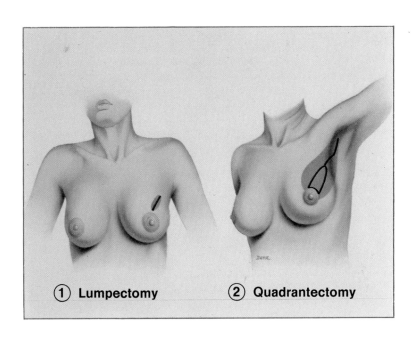

① Lumpectomy   ② Quadrantectomy

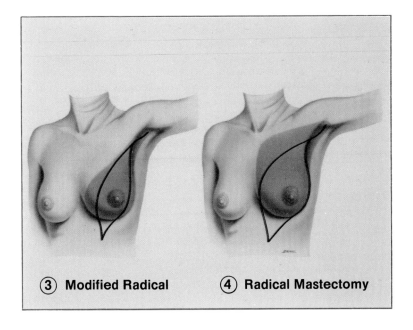

③ Modified Radical   ④ Radical Mastectomy

KIDNEYS: filtration units

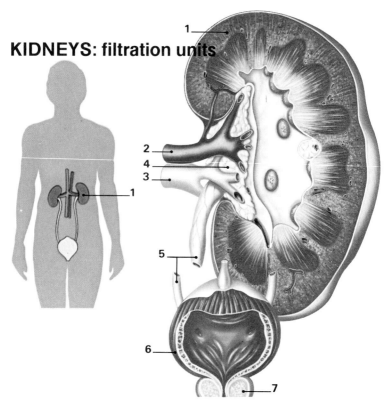

The urinary system is concerned with the formation and elimination of urine. In an adult, more than 2,500 pints of blood pass through the kidneys (**1**) each day.

Blood enters via the renal arteries (**2**) and is filtered to remove most of the waste products of metabolism. Seven pints of filtrate are produced every hour. Purified blood returns to the body circulation via the renal veins (**3**). The filtering process is carried out by more than two million tiny kidney units, or nephrons, which produce a highly concentrated solution of chemicals known as urine, which is harmful to the body if allowed to remain. Urine flows from the nephrons, first into the funnel-shaped renal pelvis (**4**) and then into the ureter (**5**).

Waves of muscular contraction passing down the ureters push the urine into the bladder (**6**). With continuous filling, the bladder, a muscular bag, expands until it holds about one pint of fluid. A circular band of muscle around the neck of the bladder, the sphincter (**7**), controls the release of urine from the body.

Mitchell Beazley Publishers, Ltd., England Atlas of the Body and Mind, Copyright © Mitchell Beazley Publishers, Ltd. 1976. Published in U.S.A. by Rand McNally & Company.

Barriers To Infection

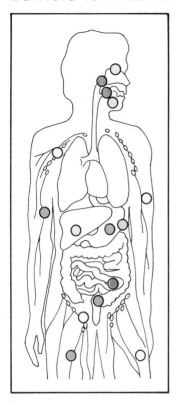

The three main routes of entry to the body for agents of disease are (**1**) through wounds, (**2**) by inhalation and (**3**) by ingestion. The skin is the first line of defense. The air we breathe is full of potentially harmful organisms but the respiratory system is designed to trap and remove any invaders. The tonsils and adenoids form a protective ring of tissue around the entrance to the throat. White blood cells in the blood and lymphatic system also fight infection.

Lachrymal glands, above the outer corner of each eye, secrete tears, which wash dust and dirt from the eyes. They contain chemicals that kill bacteria.

Tonsils and adenoids are composed of lymphoid tissue. Located at the entrances to the throat, they act as barriers to bacteria and viruses.

Salivary glands are found in the cheeks and under the tongue. The saliva they secrete contains substances which help to resist infection.

Lymph nodes are small glands which produce white blood cells. Some of these cells produce antibodies and others ingest bacteria.

The lymphatic system carries tissue fluid, or lymph, around the body. Lymph contains white cells and carries bacteria to the lymph nodes, where they are trapped and destroyed.

The liver produces some of the factors which make blood clot and so initiate wound repair.

The stomach produces hydrochloric acid, which sterilizes ingested food and kills bacteria.

The spleen, composed of lymphoid tissue, produces white blood cells and removes unwanted debris from the blood.

The small intestine is usually sterile, for bacteria have previously been killed by gastric acid and broken down by digestive enzymes.

The large intestine contains harmless bacteria which effectively exclude harmful bacteria from colonizing.

The skin is the body's main protection against disease. Invasion of organisms through the skin only occurs when it is damaged.

Mitchell Beazley Publishers, Ltd., England Atlas of the Body and Mind, Copyright © Mitchell Beazley Publishers, Ltd. 1976. Published in U.S.A. by Rand McNally & Company.

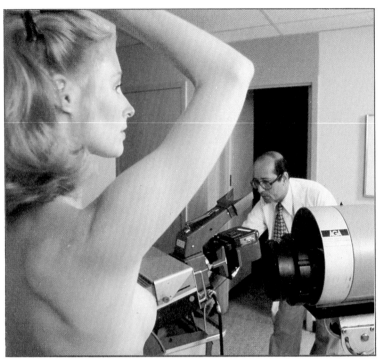

Technician examining a woman's breast with an infra-red camera. Camera detects tumors because they are warmer than the surrounding tissue.

9

CANCER OF CERVIX AND OVARIES

CERVIX CANCER

**A
Common
Cancer**

The cervix is the neck of the uterus. It is rounded and conical in shape and a portion protrudes into the vagina.

Cancer of the cervix is very common. It accounts for 25% of all Cancer found in women. It is usually seen in women between the age of 30 to 50. For some reason, not entirely known, cancer of the cervix is found much less frequently among Jewish women.

Periodic vaginal examinations is the wisest investment against developing this Cancer. There are no early warning symptoms. As the Cancer progresses, there may be bleeding after intercourse or even between periods.

TYPES OF HYSTERECTOMY

There are three types of hysterectomy: subtotal hysterectomy, total hysterectomy, and total hysterectomy with a salpingo-oophorectomy. The excised portion (which is shaded) varies in each one. In each of these procedures, however, the external genitalia and the vagina are left intact, and the woman is able to resume sexual relations.

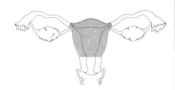

In a *subtotal hysterectomy*, all but the distal portion of the uterus is removed. The cervix is left in place. If the woman is not menopausal, she will continue to menstruate.

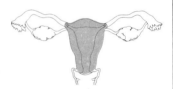

In a *total hysterectomy*, the entire uterus and the cervix are removed. This woman will no longer menstruate.

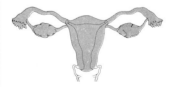

In a *total hysterectomy with a salpingo-oophorectomy*, the uterus, the cervix, the fallopian tubes, and the ovaries are removed. This woman will no longer menstruate.

**Surgery
And
Radium**

Cancer of the cervix is treated by surgery, radium or a combination. Radium capsules are inserted into the vagina and then removed after the rays have been transmitted. It is not a painful procedure. The radium remains in the genital tract from 72 to 144 hours. Your hospital stay is 2-7 days. There is some discomfort after the radium capsules are removed which is controlled by sedatives.

**Side
Effects**

There will be some disturbance in bowel function and frequency of urination. Pregnancy will no longer be possible after radium treatment and menstruation will cease.

If surgery is performed for cancer of the cervix it is generally a hysterectomy. A more extensive surgery is called an extenteration operation. This is much more radical surgery and dangerous.

OVARIAN CANCER

**Pelvic
Exams
Encouraged**

Annual pelvic examinations are the best insurance against cancer of the ovary. The ovaries (egg holder) are almond-shaped bodies attached to the uterus and lying on either side of the pelvic cavity.

If there is a malignant growth of the ovary, it is usually treated by surgical removal of all the pelvic organs. If not diagnosed early, this type of cancer tends to spread to the abdominal cavity and to distant organs.

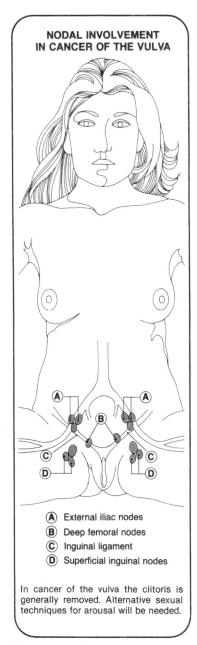

NODAL INVOLVEMENT IN CANCER OF THE VULVA

Ⓐ External iliac nodes
Ⓑ Deep femoral nodes
Ⓒ Inguinal ligament
Ⓓ Superficial inguinal nodes

In cancer of the vulva the clitoris is generally removed. Alternative sexual techniques for arousal will be needed.

The patient can get out of bed the day after surgery and the removal procedure is not dangerous nor disabling.

The ovaries secrete the sex hormones into the bloodstream. These hormones are called estrogen and progesterone. The highest incidence of Cancer of the ovary is between 40 and 50 years of age. Surgery effects a cure in about 1 out of 4 operations.

Surgery Brings Menopause

Surgical removal of the ovaries brings on a change of life (menopause). However, if one ovary alone is removed, menstruation will occur regularly and a woman can become pregnant.

10

BREAST CANCER

**Lack
Of
Nursing
A Factor**

The majority of women today do not nurse their children or, if they do, for only a short period. When organs are not put to use as nature intended, more trouble occurs. The age of *"progress"* and sophistication of many women pays a toll in disease.

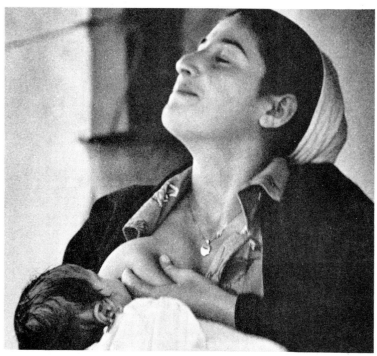

This photograph was taken near Jerusalem in 1960. The photograph reveals some of the emotional values that both mother and child enjoy through breast feeding.

**Leading
Cause
of Death**

Breast cancer accounts for one fifth of all female deaths from Cancer. It is the leading cause of death of women aged 35-54. This high incidence of breast cancer deaths in North America and Europe can, in part, be attributed to our lifestyle. During the life of a woman the female breast is involved in many abnormal activities. The breast is repeatedly subjected to fluctuations in its function and structure and it is in an exposed, unprotected position.

Any breast that has a lump should be brought to the attention of your physician. In the majority of cases a doctor can make a correct diagnosis of that lump before an operation. However, only by a biopsy can this diagnosis be made with certainty.

**Breast Cancer
Can Be Divided
Into Two
Categories
Primary and
Secondary**

Primary breast cancer is confined to the breast. Advance or secondary breast cancer is cancer that has spread to other organs. This spreading process is called metastasis.

The treatment of primary breast cancer is one in which there is much controversy. The traditional approach has been a single-stage plan in which, if the frozen section is positive, a mastectomy (removal of breast) is immediately performed. Today, many advocate a **two-stage** procedure in which the excision biopsy is followed by a decision making period as to what the definitive treatment should be when the biopsy is positive.[1]

---

[1]Stephen K. Carter, M.D., What Can You Do For Your Patients With Breast Cancer (Port Washington, New York: Medical Times), March, 1978, pp. 51, 52.

LYMPHATIC DRAINAGE
of Mammary Gland

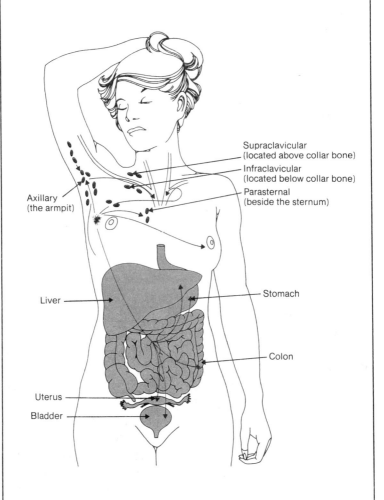

Supraclavicular
(located above collar bone)

Infraclavicular
(located below collar bone)

Parasternal
(beside the sternum)

Axillary
(the armpit)

Liver

Stomach

Colon

Uterus

Bladder

Metastasis *(movement of cancer cells)* from cancer of the mammary (breast) gland may follow several lymphatic pathways as shown above.

Two-Stage Favored

While the two-stage procedure may mean double anesthesia, it is the most widely favored. This enables the patient to arrive at a decision while awake and is less traumatic.

FOUR TYPES OF MASTECTOMIES

Lumpectomy
This is simple removal of the lump through an incision about 2" long. The operation takes 15 to 20 minutes. This is usually followed up with x-ray therapy. A woman who has had a benign breast tumor removed can breast feed her baby.

Simple
If the Cancer is confined to the breast without spread to the adjacent muscles or to the regional nodes or beyond, the breast alone is removed.

Modified radical
This procedure involves complete removal of all breast and subcutaneous tissue. Not as much chest muscles are removed as in the standard radical.

Standard radical
For many years, this was the only type of surgery used for breast cancer. This operation involves removing the breast, the two large muscles anchoring the breast to the chest wall and shoulder, and all of the lymph nodes in the armpit. This leaves considerable cosmetic defect.

There is a decline in radical mastectomies. In research done by Dr. Bernard

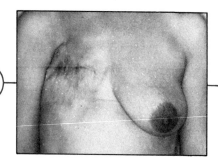

REVEALING INSIGHT

R. R. Grinker reveals some
insight into the problem one
faces with cancer:

The dread of exposing oneself
to one's spouse as
crippled, damaged, incomplete or dying
may cause
sexual inhibition or abstinence

Intimacy and sexual bodily functions
may be affected
by shame and embarrassment

Mutilation *(mastectomy)*
may make exposure and nudity
extremely painful.

There may be
an increase
in the need for contact
and reassurance . . .

On the other hand,
there may be outrage
that the partner displays
any interest in sex.[1]

---

[1] R. R. Grinker, Sex and Cancer (Medical Aspects of Human Sexuality) 1976. 10(2): 130-139.

Photograph courtesy of Sally Galbraith Thomas, R.N., Ph.D., School of Nursing, University of California.

Fisher of the University of Pittsburgh
School of Medicine they have found the
following:

In following up on
1680 breast cancer patients
for 5 years,
the results have failed to demonstrate
a significant difference in Cancer relapses
or survival
between women
who received radical mastectomy
and a carefully matched group of women
who received a more conservative
operation.

Little
Justification

Dr. Fisher believes there is little—or no—
justification for continuing to do radical
mastectomy.

SEGMENTAL MASTECTOMY

There is another new technique which is
called **segmental mastectomy.**

In segmental mastectomy,
the Cancer and surrounding tissue
are removed
along with the underarm lymph nodes,
but most of the breast remains.
In most cases
the loss of breast tissue after the operation
is barely discernible!

OTHER MEDICAL APPROACHES

There are other medical approaches in the
treatment of breast cancer.

RADIOTHERAPY

**Used
After
Surgery**

Radiotherapy involves the use of x-rays, radium, ultraviolet and other radiations. Generally it is used after mastectomy to insure that all Cancer cells are inactive. Those who undergo radiotherapy after surgery generally experience less recurrence of their Cancer, if their initial Cancer has been limited to the breast area.

CHEMOTHERAPY

**Prophylactic
Mastectomy
Not
Recommended**

The most widely used chemotherapy drug used is _doxorubicin_ (Adriamycin). This is administered intravenously. The results have not been too encouraging. More and more physicians are using various combinations of drugs in their chemotherapy procedure.

Other popular drugs include: Fluorouracil, Cytoxan and Methotrexate.

Many in orthodox medicine believe that risk of breast cancer is doubled if someone in your family has had breast cancer. As a result there has been a trend to prophylactic-mastectomy . . . that is having your breast surgically removed even though it is healthy with no sign of cancer.

Thomas K. Hunt, (University of California in San Francisco) surgery professor said . . . referring to some surgeons who perform prophylactic-mastectomy:

At some centers
plastic surgeons
who perhaps have nothing better to do
are doing hundreds of them.[1]

Dr. Patricia T. Kelly, who has a cancer-risk-counselling clinic at UCSF tells of an incident when one of her present patients was only 28 . . .

. . . she was told by a tumor board
that since three of her five sisters
were breast cancer victims,
she should have immediate bilateral
mastectomy.

HORMONE THERAPY

Temporary
Relief

Hormone therapy has been shown effective in simple Cancer problems, but only temporarily. Forms of hormone treatment include:

1. estrogen
2. androgen
3. corticosteroid therapy and
4. endocrine ablation *(removal)*.

Endocrine ablation is castration by removal of an ovary or complete hysterectomy. This sometimes prolongs life by slowing down or stopping cancer-cell division. This surgery is more effective with women who are still menstruating *(pre-menopausal)*. Estrogen therapy is the traditional approach to women more than five years post-menopause.

[1]Breast Cancer In The Family (Medical World News), June 23, 1980, p. 41.

RADIOACTIVE IMPLANTS

**Implants
Have
Degree
Of Success**

Excision of an early lesion, followed by external irradiation therapy and possibly by radioactive implants, has produced results comparable to those with extensive surgery.

The breast and regional lymph nodes are subjected to external beam irradiation, using 4 million volt x-rays. The dose is generally 5000 rads in 5 weeks. This treatment is then sometimes followed by a temporary implant of radioactive iridium-192. This implant, done under general anesthesia, delivers an additional 2000 to 3000 rads to a local area in the breast.

The implant remains in the breast for two or three days and is then removed. There are generally no side effects from this procedure except mild local discomfort. Some patients may experience a loss of appetite or occasional mild nausea or skin rash.[1]

TO THE THIRD AND FOURTH GENERATION

**We
Pass On
Poor Diets!**

At least 2 million women living today in North America will die of breast cancer. Does a woman's risk of breast cancer dou-

[1]Martin B. Levene, A New Role For Radiation Therapy, American Journal of Nursing, September, 1977, pp. 1443, 1444.

ble when there is a family history of this disease?

An Interesting Observation

It is interesting to note what the Bible says in several places including in the Old Testament book of Numbers:

> *The Lord is slow to anger*
> *and abundant in loving kindness,*
> *forgiving iniquity and transgressions;*
>
> *But He will by no means*
> *clear the guilty,*
> *visiting the iniquity of the fathers*
> *on the children*
> *to the third and fourth generations.*
> (Numbers 14:18)

Can it be that when parents ill-treat their body by eating foods that harm their bodies, they are showing disrespect for the temple of the Holy Spirit. See 1 Corinthians 6:19-20. Is it possible that the poor eating habits of past generations could be reflected in diseases in our children's children? Look at your own children. Do they reflect the eating and living habits that you follow?

11

AFTER THE MASTECTOMY

**Treat
As
Whole
Person**

When one is told that she has breast cancer, one feels very helpless and very terrified. Once the operation is over, the cancer patient wants to be treated as a whole person. She does <u>not</u> want to be told, "*Well, you look good!*"

**Approaching
Your
Husband**

There is that fear of how her husband will accept her. In losing a breast, she feels she has lost that which makes her a woman. Most husbands are mature enough to know that is not true. Let your husband in on your fears. How soon should a husband see his wife's scars? Some believe the sooner, the better. If he aids in the changing of dressings, he will feel he has a part in her recovery. He will have empathy and real understanding. Rather than breast surgery alienating your husband, it will tend to draw both of you even closer. And that closer bond will even extend to your sex life.

BREAST RECONSTRUCTION

Options Open

Choosing a prosthesis (artificial breast) can become a confusing, disappointing experience. It is not necessary to rush into buying a prosthesis. This can be done several months after the surgery. The most popular form is a liquid or silicone-filled type. These range in price from $60 to $200.

In our society, where breasts have such important symbolic and functional significance, the loss of a breast can pose adjustment problems. Many women are now seeking breast reconstruction. Not all mastectomy patients are candidates for reconstruction.

If one is considering breast reconstruction, the best time to discuss this with your surgeon is before surgery. Premastectomy consultation is extremely helpful for all concerned. It is recommended that a delay of two to six months is allowed before beginning reconstructive procedures.

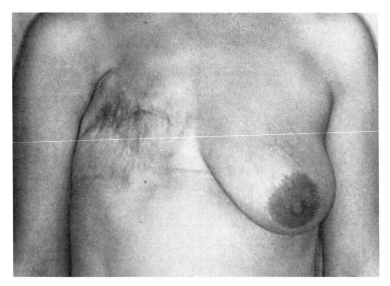

Classical Halstead radical mastectomy. Photograph illustrates unsightly scar, loss of pectoralis muscle and anterior axillary fold. Note right breast is pendulous.

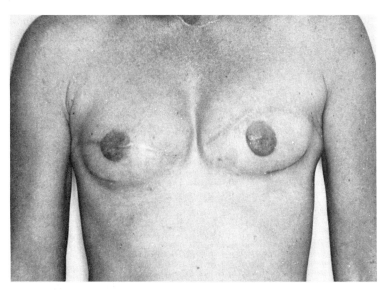

Post-operative result showing reconstructed breast mounds with simulated areolae (dark area around nipple).

Photographs courtesy of Sally Galbraith Thomas, R.N., Ph.D., School of Nursing, University of California.

**Scar
Barely
Visible**

Reconstruction surgery leaves but a barely visible scar. This surgery may consist of one operation or it may be done in several stages. A small silicone implant is inserted in the chest wall under the skin to form a "*breast mound.*" A nipple and areola *(ringlike discoloration around nipple)* can be made by sharing part of the areola from the other breast or by taking a graft from the skin of the labia *(lip of the vulva).*

1
AN M.D.'S FIGHT WITH CANCER

Anthony Sattilaro, M.D., at 48, was told he had about 18 months to live. That was June, 1978. Sattilaro had much to live for. He was a successful physician and President of Methodist Hospital in Philadelphia.

But his doctors told him his body was riddled with malignant tumors. What had started as cancer of the prostate had spread to his skull, his right shoulder, spine and ribs. The senior staff at the hospital suggested he put his house in order to prepare for his death.

In an article in the March, 1981 edition of East West Journal, Sattilaro related how surgeons attempted to keep the cancer from spreading. Three operations were performed. His left sixth rib and both of this testicles were removed. With the cancer still spreading, estrogen treatment was started. Estrogen therapy caused his weight to jump from 145 pounds to 170 pounds. The therapy caused pain and nausea. So his physicians prescribed morphine, cocaine and compazine.

By August, 1978, Dr. Sattilaro was fatigued and depressed. Coming home from his father's funeral he picked up two hitchhikers on the New Jersey Turnpike. Both were practicing the **macrobiotic diet.** They suggested to Dr. Sattilaro that such a diet could reverse his terminal cancer condition.

Sattilaro remembers:

> I just looked at him . . .
>   and thought he was just
>   some silly kid.

> Here I was a doctor
>   for twenty years.

> I knew cancer was
>   very difficult to cure,
>   and
>   we didn't have the answers.

Sattilaro hired a macrobiotic cook to prepare his meals each day. By September, 1979 his X-rays showed no more cancer left in his body. Dr. Sattilaro believes that nutrition contributed to his healing from cancer. To what extent, he will not venture a guess. Was it a combination of using orthodox medical approaches along with nutrition? Only time will tell.

To the some 1100 people who work at The Methodist Hospital in Philadelphia, Dr. Sattilaro has changed the cafeteria options so they include natural foods. The cafeteria, however, is not open to the patients themselves. At this point, Dr. Sattilaro believes it would be difficult to offer patients the option of a natural food diet.

Dr. Sattilaro has been enriched by this experience. He now looks at those who enter the hospital not as patients . . . but as people. He states:

> I understand now
>   what people go through . . .

> We are trying to get away
>   from looking at the patient
>   as a heart problem,
>   or a cancer problem . . .

> You are a person who,
>   incidentally,
>   has a problem with
>   your heart . . .
>   but you also have a family . . .
>   you may have financial problems.

> At Methodist Hospital
>   there is a real
>   caring concern
>   for the whole person.

While admitting medicine has made great strides, Dr. Sattilaro also suggests that those in orthodox medicine may have become too obsessed with the microscope and looking at diseased organs not concerned with looking at the body as a whole entity.

Orthodox medical approaches go overboard on drugs. Dr. Sattilaro does not believe the body was made to have various assortments of artificial things thrown into it. The body was meant to balance itself. While he admits he does not understand all there is to know on holistic medicine he is doing research with select patients to develop statistics on the nutritional approach to disease. While he follows a macrobiotic diet, he does not believe that this is the only diet to follow or that it is a miracle diet. Nor does he believe in the East Indian Zen Buddhism theology.

Summing up his experience, Anthony Sattilaro says:

In my past life, as an affluent American,
I would normally eat prime rib,
   potatoes with sour cream,
   and all that kind of stuff

The food was extravagant.

Now, when I go to dinner,
I see that kind of food as
poison.

I cannot believe
that God created us
to destroy these temples . . .
our bodies.

I think
He has created us
in His image
to keep our bodies
as well as possible.

Dr. Sattilaro has just published a book which centers on his remarkable recovery from cancer.

Dr. Sattilaro is still President of Methodist Hospital. The hospital is located at 2301 South Broad Street, Philadelphia, Pennsylvania 19148. Their phone number is (215) 339-5000.

The MACROBIOTIC Diet

The word "macrobiotic" means

*the art of prolonging life
as by a special diet.*

It is an outgrowth of an interpretation of Zen Buddhism introduced into the United States and Europe from Japan.

The standard macrobiotic diet consists of the following:

5-10%	Soup
25-35%	Vegetables
60%	Whole Grains

About 50% by volume cooked of every meal is whole cereal grains. This can include brown rice, barley, millet, oats, corn on the cob, corn grits, whole wheat bread or chapatis, buckwheat groats *(kasha)* rye or buckwheat noodles *(soba).*

About 25% to 35% should be vegetables. They can be steamed, boiled, baked or sauteed. However, one-third of these vegetables should be eaten raw. Commercial dressings such as mayonnaise should be avoided.

About 5% to 10% of daily food intake by volume should be a broth or miso soup. Miso soup has as its base a paste. This paste comes from naturally fermenting soy beans and barley (or wheat) for two years. Onions, carrots, cabbage, scullions and/or Chinese radish and grated ginger are cooked in a soup broth ... after which the base of miso paste is added.

Once or twice a week, the diet can include a small volume of white-meat fish.

The macrobiotic diet is a diet that avoids: meat, animal fat, poultry, dairy food, eggs, soft drinks, coffee, sugar, honey, all refined polished grains, all chemicalized foods, all hot spices or other commerical seasonings.

More information on this diet can be secured from the book, Cancer and Diet, East West Foundation, 240 Washington Street, Brookline, Massachusetts. This paperback book is $8.95.

Macrobiotic enthusiasts believe that potential cancers may be avoided and existing cancers reversed with the correct change in daily food. They believe the removing of the cancerous growth compounds the problem spreading the disease and disrupting the body balance. They suggest a macrobiotic diet as the answer. Many in the field of nutrition and orthodox medicine would disagree.

12

THE NUTRITIONAL APPROACH TO CANCER

**Nutrition
Is Vital!**

Nutrition is an excellent partner to have in your fight against cancer!

Dr. Gio Gori, who has been head of the National Cancer Institute's Diet, Nutrition and Cancer Program said:

> Physicians and med schools in general
> have not paid much attention to nutrition.
> In the past,
> much of the information about nutrition
> in the therapy of disease
> was based on faith
> and not necessarily on experiments
> that were scientifically reproducible.[1]

It is not unusual for malnutrition to be a secondary cause of death in cancer patients.

---

[1]Robert A. Becker, Nutrition Fights Cancer, (New York: National Observer), June 27, 1977, pp. 1, 15.

VITAMIN A

**Blocks
Formation
Of
Cancer Cells**

A deficiency of Vitamin A may lead to the development of cancer. Vitamin A's cancer-preventing potential may be its control of a process called cell differentiation.

Differentiation allows the cell to carry out its normal functions. Scientists in Japan found evidence of a connection between Vitamin A deficiency and cancer in a 10-year study of 122,261 men aged 40 and above. These men had a low intake of green and yellow vegetables (It is these vegetables that are high in Vitamin A). They were noted for a high incidence of prostate cancer deaths.

It is believed that Vitamin A interferes and blocks the formation of cancer cells within the body.

Vitamin A has been shown to boost the immune response of patients with inoperable lung cancer (Oncology, vol. 34, 1977).

**Richest
Source**

Beef liver is the richest source of Vitamin A found in a food. Vitamin A, like Vitamins D and E are fat-soluble vitamins. This means it is not excreted in the urine. (like water-soluble vitamins) but stored in the body for further use. Most natural Vitamin A supplements are derived from fish or shark liver oil.

The Recommended Dietary Allowance for

Vitamin A is 5,000 I.U. for adults. Some nutritionists believe that doses of 20,000 I.U. daily should be harmless. Symptoms of Vitamin A toxicity include:

itching dry skin
headache
hair loss
aching bones

Here are some foods that are rich in Vitamin A:

	Vitamin A I.U.
Beef Liver (1/4 lb.)	5,100
Beet Greens (1 cup)	5,100
Broccoli (1 cup)	3,750
Carrots (1 cup diced/steamed)	15,750
Collards (1 cup/steamed)	15,600
Mustard Greens (1 cup/steamed)	8,120
Raw Papaya	7,000
Watermelon (1 4" x 8" wedge)	5,458

Energy Builder

Desiccated liver has been claimed by nutritionists to be a cancer preventive. It can also detoxify cortisone and thyroid hormone, eliminating the distressing side effects. It is an energy builder and is especially important for the elderly, who tire easily.

Desiccated liver is concentrated beef liver in powder or tablet form, which has been dried in a vacuum at a low temperature to retain its nutrient values. It is rich in Vitamins A, C, and D and also in iron, calcium, phosphorus and copper.

**The
Lymph Gland
And
Vitamins
A and C**

Many Cancers eventually invade lymph glands, where a fluid called lymph is stored. These glands drain the fluid from various parts of the body into the veins. The lymphatic system plays an important part in protecting the body against many diseases, including Cancer.

Growing Cancers have a way of invading the lymph glands and destroying them. The drug prednisolone has the power of reducing the activity of lymph glands and produces a short-term remission of cancerous lymph glands and lymphatic leukemias. But it has side effects which undermine the body's overall resistance to Cancer. Some scientists believe that a combination of Vitamin A with C and prednisolone can produce a promising effect.

Colonics

Some nutritionists believe colon irrigation can be beneficial to those suffering from cancer. They suggest that a build-up of toxic wastes on the colon walls can eventually cause a back-up of poisons through the body. The next four pages describe colonic therapy.

1
ALL ABOUT COLONICS

A **colonic irrigation** involves injecting into the colon a large amount of water, <u>flowing in and out at constant intervals.</u>

This continuous flowing in and flowing out washes out material situated above the defecation area and washes the walls of the colon as high as water can be made to reach. Colonics use 20-30 gallons of water — but only a pint or two at a time. A colon irrigation takes one-half to one hour.

Generally, a series of 6-12 colonics are given to remove the encrustations of the colon and empty out the pockets.

A majority of minerals are assimilated in the colon. If the colon is not functioning at normal levels, the body can become mineral-poor and illness will occur.

Many people have parasites in their colon. It was believed that parasites rob the body of nutrients. The main problem, colonic specialists believe, is the excreta the parasites eject from their body (while in your colon). Such poisons can affect a person's disposition, making him nervous and irritable, unable to cope with each day's problems.

Those specialists who practice colonic irrigation say that colon problems are not simply problems of the elderly. One colonic therapist recalled a case of a 5-year-old boy who was constipated since birth. As a result of his constipation his colon was extended or elongated making for longer transit time. He had a variety of symptoms. He had skin eruptions, was hyperactive and had digestive problems.

There are very few qualified colonic therapists in the United States. They are generally concentrated in high population areas such as Los Angeles, Miami, New York and Chicago.

Depression, nervousness, irritability, frequent crying spells, fatigue and severe constipation are symptoms which suggest a distressed colon. Upon X-ray it is not unusual to find parts of the colon double the size it should be. An area of such a colon can also be filled with parasites. The colon in such an individual can also be elongated and rise high into the diaphragm, causing chest pains. It can mimic a heart attack . . . when gas is present in this colon area. In such cases one colonic treatment is not considered sufficient. Many colonic therapists would recommend 6-10 treatments over a short period of time.

Many people think that only meat eaters can develop parasites. But even vegetarians can get parasites into their body. Parasites can enter vegetables from the fertilizer that is used in farming. Parasites can enter the skin of someone walking barefoot. There need not be a scratch on the foot. They can enter through the pores in the feet.

Diverticulitis is another problem with which some colonic thera-pists have good success. Many who have advance cases of diver-ticulitis believe colonic irrigation is a better first alternative to a colos-tomy operation. These little sacs (diverticuli) appear on the colon where there is a weak area and accumulate waste material. In colonic therapy, the water washes the affected area.

In **oxygen-colonics.** ... along with water, a carefully regulated amount of oxygen is also introduced into the colon. While the water does its job of washing the colon, the oxygen, therapists say, heals the infected area. Medically speaking, diverticuli are a problem you have to live with the rest of your life. Colonic therapists would dis-agree. Many believe they can heal this condition.

Colonic therapists seek to cleanse the entire colon with water over a period of several treatments. When successful they can remove fe-cal encrustations that have lodged in the colon for many, many years. As this putrefied material flushes out, the stench is very strong. It rapidly conveys to the patient how clogged up his system had become.

With a clogged colon often a person will have liver problems. The reason: the liver will pass on its waste into the colon. With a poorly functioning colon, often these poisons cannot get through initially and back up into the liver again.

One colonic therapist reports that 50-60% of the patients he sees have tapeworms and 80% of the patients have some form of para-sites. Tapeworms can be 20 feet long in your colon and as thick as your thumb.

Some would argue that colonics *(intestinal irrigations)* do harm by removing normal mucus and by producing colitis. Nutritionists who understand colonic therapy would disagree. Foul, putrefactive masses lodged on colon walls do not contain normal mucus and in themselves would encourage colitis. Therefore, a series of colonics would be deemed highly beneficial to restoring health.

A colonic is not a cure-all. If the individual does not correct his dietary habits the same conditions can recur.

A series of colonic irrigations, therapists suggest, removes practically the whole fecal contents of the colon, softens and removes the large masses of mucus present in mucous colitis and restores the colon to its normal size. Such treatment, they believe, can improve the health conditions of those with arthritis, rheumatism, neuritis and a host of other diseases.

One indication that colon therapy is needed, according to Dr. Cora Smith King is the appearance on the chest, abdomen and back of bright red mole-like spots. These are called little _hemangiomas_ (blood vessel tumors) or _telangiectasia_ (end vessel dilation). Dr. Smith suggests these little hemangiomas are tiny danger flags, signifying intestinal toxemia.[1]

Colonic irrigations were popular many years ago and administered even in hospitals until the late 1950's. Much of the data on colonic therapy was written by medical doctors.

W.A. Bastedo in a Journal of American Medical Association publication reported:

> ... colon irrigations are employed in chronic states of the bowel, such as are encountered in mucous colitis, intestinal putrefactive toxemia and in cases in which a focus of infection is believed to reside in the bowel, as in certain cases of rheumatism, neuritis, secondary anemias ...[2]

Today, colonic irrigations are given by colonic therapists or nurses. They are, as a rule, not available in hospitals but rather in natural health clinics. Some are run in conjunction with chiropractic services. They are generally listed in the yellow pages of the phone books under _Colonic Irrigation._ Check with your doctor.

---

[1]Joseph E.G. Waddington, M.D. Scientific Intestinal Irrigation and Adjuvant Therapy (Chicago: The Bryan Publishers) 1940, p. 28.

[2]W.A. Bastedo, Colon Irrigation (Chicago: Journal of American Medical Association, Council on Physical Therapy) 1932, February 27, 98:734.

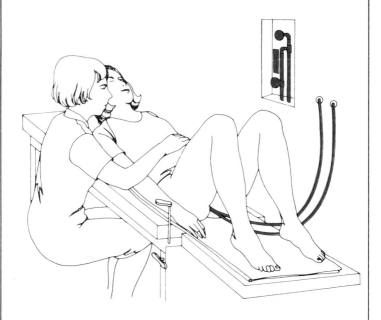

Colonic therapists suggest <u>five</u> ways colonic irrigations are beneficial:

1. Removes practically the whole fecal contents of the colon.
2. Cleanses the delicate mucous membrane of protozoa, bacteria and inflammatory products.
3. Gives valuable information obtainable from the stool concerning physical well-being of patient.
4. Softens and moves the large masses of mucus present in mucous colitis.
5. Removes odors of fermentation and putrefaction.

Colon therapy is a purely physical process of detoxification. Therapists believe, when properly given, the poisonous matter is quickly and completely removed from the <u>entire</u> colon. Many gallons of water are injected into the colon in a steady flow <u>in</u> and <u>out</u> of the colon, thus breaking up the impaction, gently and painlessly.

VITAMIN B COMPLEX

**Acts
As An
Inhibitor**

All B vitamins are water-soluble. Basically, the B Complex range of vitamins provide the body with energy by converting carbohydrates into glucose, which the body "burns" to produce energy. They are vital in the metabolism of fats and protein, and are considered the single most important factor for health of the nerves. Becaue B vitamins are water-soluble, any excess is excreted in the urine. Therefore, they must be continually replaced.

One of the differences between a normal cell and a cancer cell is that the normal cell contains an inhibitor of a certain enzyme involved in protein systhesis and cell reproduction, while the cancer cell does not. That <u>inhibitor</u> has been identified as **Vitamin B$_3$** (Nicotinamide).[1]

**Produce
Lecithin**

<u>Inositol</u> is another part of the Vitamin B complex that is considered beneficial in anti-cancer therapy. Researchers have also found it beneficial in treating diabetics and those with high cholesterol levels. Inositol is effective in promoting the body's production of <u>lecithin</u>. Caffeine may create an inositol shortage in the body.

[1]Food Supplements Against Cancer, (Emmaus, Pennsylvania: *Prevention*), July, 1972, pp. 138-149.

**Take
Together**

For the most part, the B-complex Vitamins are dependent upon one another for their interrelation. An inadequate intake of one may impair the utilization of others. It is unwise to take large amounts individually of one B-complex Vitamin because it can cause a B-complex imbalance. The need for the B-complex Vitamins increases during infection or stress. Sugar and alcohol destroy the B-complex Vitamins.

IS LAETRILE AN OPTION?

**Is
Laetrile
Beneficial?**

Vitamin B_{17} (Laetrile) is a highly controversial compound. Dr. Ernest Krebs, Sr. was the first to use laetrile therapeutically in the United States. He called it Vitamin B_{17}. Many in orthodox medicine consider Laetrile to be highly toxic due to the cyanide in the chemistry of this vitamin. Others like Dr. Dean Burk, chief cytologist of the National Cancer Institute state that:

> Laetrile is remarkably non-toxic . . .
> compared with virtually
> all cancer chemotherapeutic agents
> currently studied.[1]

Nutrition Almanac reports that natural cyanide is locked in a sugar molecule and is normally found in over 2000 known unrefined foods and grasses. Sprouting seeds produce from 30 to 50 times as

[1]Laetrile—An Answer To Cancer? (Emmaus, Pennsylvania: *Prevention*), December 1971, p. 162.

much B_{17} as does the mature plant. Shell-
ed and unshelled apricot kernels contain 2
to 3% amygdalin. Laetrile is an
amygdalin.[1]

**Highly
Selective**

Advocates of laetrile say it is a highly selective substance that attacks only the
cancerous cells. It causes an enzyme
called rhodanese to detoxify the cyanide,
which is then excreted through the urine.
Cancer cells, however, are deficient in
rhodanese. They instead are surrounded
by another enzyme, beta-glucosidase. This
releases the bound cyanide from the laetrile at the site of malignancy. Thus advocates believe that laetrile attacks only the
malignant areas.

**Richest
Sources**

The richest sources of nitrilosides (aside
from apricots) are the wild crabapple, the
market cranberry, red and black raspber-
ries, blackberries and huckleberries. Also
on this list are wild grasses such as white
clover, lupine and wheat grass.

Lentils are very high in nitrilosides, when
sprouted, as are lima beans. Grains high in
nitrilosides are millet, buckwheat and the
flax family . . . also cassava, the bread of
the tropics. Sorghum cane is high in nitrilosides; sugar cane and the sugar made
from it have none!

Sprouting seeds, alfalfa, mung beans, lentils have as much as 50 times or more ni-
triloside content than in the mature plant.

[1]John D. Kirschmann, Nutrition Almanac, (New
York: McGraw-Hill Book Company), 1975, pp. 35, 36.

VITAMIN C

Dr. Ewan Cameron, chief surgeon of a 440-bed hospital in Scotland, uses high doses of Vitamin C and is obtaining some encouraging results.

In an interview in *Prevention* magazine, Dr. Cameron reports that in giving Vitamin C to some very advanced Cancer patients, the first few patients responded very remarkably.

In 1973, Dr. Cameron began treatment on a truck driver who was pronounced terminally ill with reticulum cell sarcoma *(cancer cells in lymph nodes and other tissues)*. A therapy was started of 10 grams of Vitamin C intravenously for 10 days, then 10 grams per day orally thereafter. Within 10 days, appetite returned, night sweats had ceased and his enlarged liver and spleen shrank to normal size.

When the daily dose of Vitamin C was steadily reduced . . . the Cancer symptoms returned. When the Vitamin C program was renewed, the symptoms disappeared. He then took maintenance doses of 12.5 grams per day thereafter. Six years later he was still doing well.[1]

Dr. Cameron believes the way to control Cancer's invasion into the body cells is to

---

[1] Dominick Bosco, Vitamin C and Cancer, (Emmaus, Pennsylvania: *Prevention*), November, 1975, pp. 152-57; July, 1979, pp. 48-55.

stop them by way of a substance called *hyaluronidase inhibitor.* By 1971 he was fairly sure that Vitamin C *(ascorbic acid)* was required for the body's synthesis of this inhibitor.

Live Longer

He has found that 90% of the terminally ill Cancer patients live significantly longer than could be otherwise expected . . . and about 10% live a remarkably long time with Vitamin C.

It is believed by some nutritionists that Vitamin C stimulates the immune system of the body.

Encouraging Report

Dr. Linus Pauling believes that the incidence and mortality from Cancer could be decreaed by 75% by the proper use of Vitamin C alone. Dr. Pauling cites a case of a woman with a brain tumor who was paralyzed because of it. She was scheduled for an operation and she was warned the paralysis would become worse. She refused the operation, began taking 15 grams of Vitamin C a day. Two months later the brain scan could not pick up the tumor and her paralysis was gone.

As therapeutic insurance, Dr. Cameron takes 3 grams of Vitamin C every morning.

Bladder Cancer

Bladder cancer kills over 10,000 Americans a year. Nutritionists believe that Vitamin C can keep bladder cancer from recurring. The key is to take enough Vitamin C so that the excess spills over into the urine. Alcohol, soft drinks, coffee and nicotine are contributory factors in bladder cancer.

VITAMIN E

Lowers Level of Free Radicals

Researchers from the Cleveland Clinic Foundation have found that Vitamin E, Vitamin C and the mineral selenium all markedly reduce the injuries wrought by Cancer-causing chemicals upon the structure of living human chromosomes.[1]

Vitamin E is believed to be the most potent natural antioxidant. Free radicals are atoms having an odd number of electrons. This makes them extremely unstable. It is believed they play a key role in triggering the development of Cancer. The theory is that Vitamin E lowers the level of free radical reactions in humans.

A woman who had very painful lumps in her breasts was diagnosed as fibrosis and a mastectomy was suggested. She, instead, began taking 600 I.U. of Vitamin E three times a day and experienced absence of pain and no lumps, according to a July, 1977 report on page 174 of *Prevention*.

Vitamin E has been used by some to offset the side effects of radiation and chemotherapy.

---

[1]Marco Bruno, Better Nutrition for Less Cancer (Emmaus, Pennsylvania: *Prevention*), September, 1973, pp. 63-71.

1
The BRENNAN Approach to Cancer

Dr. Richard O. Brennan is both a physician and surgeon. He has been awarded the following certificates by the medical profession: Doctor of Osteopathic Medicine, Doctor of Medicine, Doctor of Public Health, Graduate Pharmacist. He was Medical Director of the Bellevue Metabolic Clinic of Houston, Texas.

Dr. Brennan is presently Medical Director of the Brennan Preventive Medical Center in Houston, Texas.

His book, <u>Coronary? Cancer? God's Answer: Prevent It!</u> begins with the following:

> Many of today's men of medicine
> are beginning to believe
> that our present sick-care system
> is headed for a catastrophic breakdown . . .
>
> We must not be fooled
> by the tendency of
> scientific researchers
> to look at one part of the body
> and think they will find the answer to cancer
> in one area.
>
> Cancer is not a local disease,
> and the malignancy epidemic
> cannot be solved
> by the microscopic study
> of the structures of abnormal tissues.
> Cancer is a disease that affects
> the entire body
> and must be considered
> as a total body problem . . .
>
> We have overlooked
> the interaction of
> spirit, mind and body . . .
>
> We have reached such a state
> of pseudoscientific sophistication
> that we will not accept
> the empirical approach[1]
> that can save our lives and
> prevent the high cost of our sick-care system.

---

[1]**empirical approach:** *relying on practical experience without reference to scientific principles or theory.*

Dr. Brennan concludes by stating:

> Peace of mind
> does not come in capsules.
> Peace of mind
> comes from the inner qualities
> that are based on the
> soundness of body and mind
> that is in tune with God.
>
> There is more
> power in prayer
> than in
> a medical prescription.[1]

In 1977, Dr. Brennan's daughter discovered she had cancer. In Houston, doctors told her she had an *"Oat Cell"* cancer of the hilium (the opening where vessels enter) of the left lung. They suggested chemotherapy. She returned to Kansas City and began some chemotherapy and radiation treatments.

Dr. Brennan was concerned for he knew the radiation would make her very sick. He noticed a research report on <u>SOD</u> *(superoxide dismutase).*[2] Dr. Brennan's daughter, Phyllis, already had three radiation treatments and was feeling the side effects. The SOD was given to her in liquid form after this series and the radiation sickness did not recur.

Phyllis was placed on an overall nutrition program which included <u>protomorphagens</u> *(substances made from basic tissues)* as well as a microemulsion of A-E and enzymes. Two years later Phyllis was completely negative for cancer findings.

It was Nobel Prize Laureate Albert Szent-Gyorgyi who said:

> Very few people
> know what real health is
> because most are occupied
> with killing themselves slowly.

To which Dr. Brennan adds:

> Our cancer research is
> misdirected, inefficient and inadequate.

---

[1]Richard O. Brennan, D.O., M.D., <u>Coronary? Cancer? God's Answer: Prevent It</u> (Eugene, Oregon: Harvest House, Publishers) 1979, pp. 7, 9, 10.
[2]Largely through Dr. Brennan's efforts, this enzyme is now on the market in tablet form under the name of <u>Dismuzyne.</u>

3
The BRENNAN Approach to Cancer

We have
as many people living off the disease
as are dying from it.

The government spends
billions on cancer research,
but at the same time
allows known carcinogens
in our processed foods,
subsidizes cigarettes,
and continues to develop
new radiation,
surgical and chemotherapy techniques
when burning, cutting and poisoning
have already proved
largely unsuccessful.[1]

Dr. Brennan explains that each individual has two kinds of metabolism in his body.

1. *Anabolic* **metabolism**

    This is the build-up phase. Children, because they are constantly growing, are in the *anabolic* phase.

    As we grow older, we are supposed to be in a metabolic balance; that is, not breaking down any more than we are building up daily.

2. *Catabolic* **metabolism**

    This is the break-down state. Dr. Brennan explains that this is where we get the term *"break-down diseases"* or chronic, degenerative diseases.

The great tragedy is that too large a percentage of Americans are not rebuilding and repairing what they break down daily. Out of metabolic balance, they are in a catabolic stage and thus become ill.

Dr. Brennan is a firm believer in the proposition that if you correct the nutritional deficiencies that exist in your body, you will see a difference. Your aging process will slow down. Your virility and vitality will be renewed. You will become more agile. Dr. Brennan believes:

Degenerative diseases
are not caused by

---

[1] Ibid., p. 71.

viruses, bacteria or parasites,
but by the body's
inadequate metabolic response
to a condition
in which the cells of the body
are being slowly poisoned
by too many wrong things or
by not getting enough
of the right things
at the right time.[1]

Dr. Brennan emphasizes the need for understanding how the enzymes function in our body. He states that life is largely the result of biochemical reactions and that these reactions depend entirely upon the catalyzing effect of enzymes.[2].

Enzymes break down our food material so that food can be assimilated and become available for cell utilization. They enhance a chemical reaction, speeding it up. But the enzyme, amazingly remains unchanged at the end of this interaction. It is available for its next task over and over again.

Enzymes need assistance in this service to the body function. That assistance comes in the form of *coenzymes*. Among coenzymes are *vitamins*. This is why, Dr. Brennan believe, vitamins are so essential to the diet.

Cancer robs the body of nutrients. Vitamins and minerals are essential to insure that the enzyme system is in a fully functional state. SOD *(superoxide dismutase)* is what Dr. Brennan used on his daughter. SOD is an enzyme which prevents the destructive effects of superozide.

Dr. Brennan pays tribute to the late Dr. Max B. Gerson as a man *"far ahead of the times."* Dr. Gerson believed that the source of immunity was a healthy functioning digestive tract, particularly the liver. Gerson's diet was directed to cleansing the patient's liver of its accumulated poisons and building a health program through a proper selection of nutrients.

---

[1]Ibid., p. 93.

[2]Enzymes are catalysts . . . the essential biological catalysts that make life possible. We live because our bodies contain thousands of different kinds of enzymes that regulate our life processes.

Dr. Brennan states that a healthy body is kept in metabolic balance by four main factors:

1. Healthy nutrition and digestion.
2. Healthy elimination.
3. Healthy physical activity.
4. Healthy mental attitude.[1] (a positive attitude free of fear)

Dr. Brennan's book, in his last three chapters, suggests diet and other considerations he feels helpful in finding the answer to not only heart disease and cancer but other ailments. One of these last chapters on Cell Assurance presents a program *"to give you a disease-free life full of vim and vigor."*

Dr. Richard O. Brennan's book is titled: <u>Coronary? Cancer? God's Answer: Prevent It!</u> It is published by Harvest House Publishers.

---

[1] Ibid., p. 165.

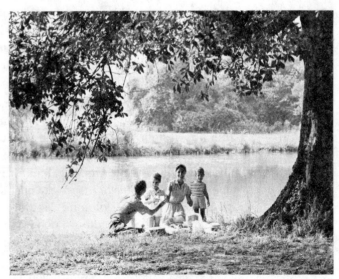

A relaxed, healthy attitude is essential.

13

FIGHTING CANCER WITH MINERALS

MAGNESIUM

**Aids
Immunization
System**

Magnesium is very important to the body's metabolism. Magnesium plays a part in at least 30 different enzymatic reactions and is concerned mostly with the regulation of growth, metabolism and division of cells, according to Dr. George M. Hass, a Chicago pathologist.[1]

It is believed that a magnesium deficiency leads to a breakdown of the body's natural immune system. Magnesium and calcium are closely related. You should be getting about 2½ to 2¾ times more calcium than magnesium in order to insure the best use of both minerals. Dolomite is the best source of this combination. Foods rich in magnesium include whole grains, spinach, corn and nuts as well as peas, lima beans, beet greens and collard leaves.

[1] Michael Clark, Leukemia, Immunity and Magnesium, (Emmaus, Pennsylvania: Prevention), July, 1975, pp. 56-61.

SELENIUM

Is
This
Part of
The
Answer?

Dr. Gerhard Schrauzer, professor of chemistry at the University of California at San Diego suggests that the higher the selenium intake the lower the Cancer mortality rate in the common types of Cancer—stomach, leukemia, large intestine, rectum, pancreas, lung, breast, uterus and prostate.

He further reports that the average American diet contains only 50 to 150 mcg. of selenium. (Note: that's micrograms, *not milligrams.*) He estimates that people must have between 200 to 300 micrograms of selenium a day for maximum Cancer protection.[1]

Selenium is a trace mineral. It is found in bran and germ of cereals, in vegetables such as broccoli, onions, and tomatoes. It is also found in tuna. Selenium is a natural antioxidant and works closely with Vitamin E. Too much selenium can be toxic. Brewer's yeast is, perhaps, the best single day-to-day supplement to make sure you not only get selenium in your diet but absorb it and put it to work.

[1]Paul Martin, Is There An Anti-Cancer Diet?, (Los Angeles, Calif: *Let's Live*), August, 1980, pp. 57-62.

1
The MINERAL Approach To Illness
An Interview with Paul Eck

Dr. Paul Eck has a degree in the field of naprapathy. Naprapathy is a system of therapy which attributes all disease to disorders of the nervous system, ligaments and connective tissue.

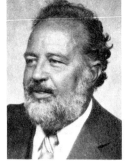

He is director of Analytical Research Laboratories in Phoenix, Arizona which specializes in interpreting hair tests. Paul Eck prepares vitamin and mineral programs for many medical doctors and other health practitioners.

Dr. Eck has very definite views on how to correct basic illnesses. They differ quite dramatically from the standard medical approach to disease. In fact, they differ also from many of the usual nutritional approaches to disease, as well!

Dr. Eck believes that much of what is going on today in the field of nutrition is guesswork. Too many people are spending anywhere from $5000 to $15,000 to correct health deficiencies and are no better off physically. The problem, as Eck sees it, is that it is not the products they are taking that are wrong . . . but that the necessary knowledge and application to utilize these various nutrients is missing!

In an interview with Sam and Loren Biser of The Healthview Newsletter, Eck commented:

> It's not the amount of vitamins that you take nor is it the amount of minerals you are taking or anything else . . . the products or the money that you are spending . . . I think a lot of this is pure waste because if it is not being applied in a scientific way there's no way that it's ever going to work![1]

---

[1]Paul Eck, Your Minerals and Your Health (To secure this one hour cassette, send $10 direct to Healthview Newsletter, Box 6670, Charlottesville, Virginia 22906)

Other cassettes by Dr. Paul Eck on various metabolic dysfunctions and philosophy of health are available from Analytical Research Laboratories, Inc., 2338 West Royal Palm Road, Suite F, Phoenix, Arizona 85021.

When Paul Eck first became interested in hair analysis he discovered he had a low zinc level of 9 (the normal zinc level is 20). He also had hypoglycemia, he was nervous and had a tendency towards diabetes. He also knew his anxiety levels were high.

To try and correct his low zinc level he began taking 3 zinc tablets a day. He was surprised to find that he did not get better. In fact, he became worse and experienced extreme fatigue. He decided to go off the zinc and his energy level began to come back to what it was before.

Simply adding zinc to your system can cause other problems. Too much zinc has a tendency to make your copper level low. The normal level for copper in the human body, according to Eck, is 2.5mg./% He states that anyone with a copper level of 1.0 is in a potential cancerous state.

Low copper levels symptoms may show up as: fatigue, anemia, joint pain and depression. Eck believes this can lead to a cancerous condition because:

> ... the copper inside the cell regulates the respiratory oxidation mechanism which prevents you from getting cancer.[1]

Paul Eck also says that if one has a high copper level ... and takes a multiple vitamin/mineral tablet or supplement that has copper in it, their physical problem will become worse. The additional copper, adding to their already high level, will accentuate their illness and the other vitamins and minerals in the daily supplement will be of no value. The indiscriminate taking of vitamins and minerals can be a hit and miss type of therapy. It can be a total waste of money, according to Eck. He believes that up to 90% of the people taking multiple vitamin supplements are damaging their health.

Eck states that copper is the most dangerous of all the required minerals, if you are not aware of what your body requires. Simply to take copper supplements on a guess-basis can be hazardous to your health.

---

[1]Ibid.

Paul Eck also believes that excessive Vitamin C taken over a considerable length of time and in certain "biological types" can cause cancer. He suggests that soils that are high in calcium and magnesium protect against cancer. Any mineral, therefore, that can lower these two minerals (calcium and magnesium) or copper can cause a cancerous condition.

In a recorded interview for <u>The Healthview Newsletter,</u> Eck stated:

> There is no question that a person can take Vitamin C
> in some cancer cases and derive results.
>
> But, just as zinc lowers copper, which is perhaps the most
> protective mineral against cancer . . . Vitamin C also has
> a copper lowering effect, and over the years, can cause
> cancer.[1]

Dr. Paul Eck does not believe it is necessary in the majority of cases to give large doses of Vitamin C. He says that copper makes up a part of an enzyme called <u>ascorbic acid oxidase.</u> An <u>oxidase</u> is a catalyst. It is the copper in this formula that activates the enzyme. If this ascorbic acid oxidase enzyme is missing, Eck believes then that Vitamin C cannot be oxidized to adequate amounts in the body. Therefore, Eck concludes, if this optimal oxidation is not taking place, large amounts of Vitamin C are not only useless but can initiate various disease proccesses.

If your body is not functioning properly, the vitamins will not excrete the excess minerals you may be taking in your daily supplements. Instead they accumulate in the body. If your body is deficient in Vitamin B[6], as an example, you will have a tendency to accumulate copper in the body. This can result in a <u>toxic</u> level of <u>copper</u> in your system.

Dr. Eck does not encourage the taking of multiple vitamins and minerals. He feels this indiscrimate use is detrimental to one's health . . . since every individual is biochemically different.

---

[1]Ibid.

Paul Eck is a firm believer in using hair analysis tests. The reason, he states:

> *A hair analysis test is the only method developed that has any validity at all as far as measuring what actually is occurring in the tissues of the body.*
>
> *It has the benefit of being able to give you a metabolic pattern of every metabolic activity that is occurring in your body over a period of time.*[1]

Dr. Eck believes that blood tests, in this context, are frequently invalid because they give you an up-to-the-minute readout. It is not a true reflection of what is happening in the tissues over a period of time. A person taking a high amount of Vitamin C could be releasing from his system large amounts of cholesterol. If a blood test were taken at that time it would show a high cholesterol level. However, what the physician does not realize is that it is not a build-up of cholesterol but, quite the opposite, a beneficial flushing of cholesterol out of the body.

Too many people, Dr. Eck suggests, take maganese when they have a manganese deficiency . . . they take iron when they have an iron deficiency, etc. **This is wrong.** To give iron to raise iron is to lower iron!

Dr. Louis Kervan, in his book, Biological Transmutations makes the following observations:

> For IRON deficiency . . . give Manganese.
> For MANGANESE deficiency . . . give Copper.
> For MAGNESIUM deficiency . . . give Zinc.
> For ZINC deficiency . . . give Magnesium.

---

[1]Ibid.

When you go on a correct vitamin/ mineral supplementation, the excess minerals and toxic minerals (such as cadmium, lead, aluminum) will start to unload and flush out of your system. This unloading will cause headaches and numerous other symptoms which will vary with the toxic metal or combination of toxic metals being eliminated, and in some cases make you feel worse. This is a natural occurrence as your body gets rid of these unwanted elements to get you on the road to full recovery.

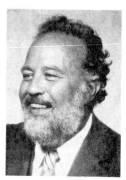

Dr. Eck believes that mineral imbalances should be corrected mainly by using <u>small</u> potency vitamins and minerals. He says it just takes a very small amount of a mineral to initiate a major physiological process in the body. Any amount over that, he states, will cause exactly the opposite reaction.

Paul Eck believes that mineral therapy is also indirectly hormone therapy. Through the results found in hair analysis he has been able to see people go off hormone therapy, estrogen, even off of thyroxin. He has used manganese and copper to improve their thyroid function where indicated.

Paul Eck is very familiar with Diabetes. His grandmother, his mother was diabetic. He and his brother were pre-diabetic. Dr. Eck states he can determine from a hair analysis, years in advance, whether a person will become a diabetic.

Paul Eck says that 90% of the people who have diabetes have more than enough insulin circulating in their blood. When you have a low calcium to magnesium ratio (such as 3.3 to 1) you have an individual that has diabetes. And if the ratio is high, such as <u>10</u> parts calcium to <u>1</u> part magnesium . . . you are in the diabetic area.[1]
Eck states:

> *One problem in about 10% of the diabetics is the lack of calcium in the pancreas. This condition results in an inability of the Islets of Langerhans to secrete insulin . . .*

---

[1] The calcium to magnesium <u>ratio</u> normally is 6.7 to 1. This means for every 1 part of magnesium in your system, you should have 6.7 parts of calcium.

because when the calcium drops below a certain level you can't even initiate the secretion of the insulin that is manufactured and is being stored in pancreatic Islets of Langerhans tissue.

So what you have to do is, by one means or another, raise the calcium level back up to a close to normal ratio between the magnesium and then you automatically get a secretion of insulin.

This occurs in your insulin-deficiency diabetics ... which only accounts for about 10 or 12% of the cases.

Dr. Eck states that the rest of the problem in diabetes lies either in the transport of the insulin to the cell itself or, when it gets to the cell, there is a lack of a receptor at the cell site on the cell membrane. Those receptors are all minerals! Therefore, Dr. Eck concludes:

If the proper mineral is not available in the body for transport of the insulin to the cell ... it doesn't get there in the first place.

Secondly, even when it gets there, if some receptor is not present, and there are multiple receptors on the cell membrane ... then, of course, the insulin can't even enter the cell and do what it is supposed to do!

We have had such great reports especially in diabetes.

You know the old saying that says "Once you've been on insulin, you're going to stay on it the rest of your life ..." that's the same statement they use for hypothyroidism. They say: "Once you're on thyroid, you're going to be on it forever. Make up your mind to it."

Some individuals have been able to have their insulin requirement reduced or completely eliminated within a few weeks. These, of course, are spectacular cases. There are also insulin-taking diabetics who require a year or two to bring about a complete correction. The individual must be extremely cooperative. Attempts to correct diabetes must be done under the supervision of a doctor.

Dr. Eck says that those taking oral hypoglycemic agents for diabetics are the easiest cases to correct. Correcting those with juvenile diabetes is much more difficult ... unless the individual faithfully stays on the health program.

Dr. Eck believes there are 7 mineral clues as to whether a person is developing cancer. The more of these clues they have the more severe their condition is. Here are the clues:

*1. Calcium/Magnesium ratio of less than 2 parts of calcium to 1 part of magnesium . . . is a cancer indicator.

*2. Calcium/Magnesium ratio of over 14 parts of calcium to 1 part of magnesium . . . is a cancer indicator.

*3. Sodium/Potassium inversion. Normally sodium is 25 in ratio to your potassium, which is 10. This is a 2.5 to 1 sodium to potassium ratio. If the ratio inverts (goes lower than 1.5 to 1) this could be indicative of cancer, kidney disease, hypertension, infections, osteoarthritis, etc.!

*4. Zinc/copper ratio of over 16 parts of zinc to 1 part of copper . . . is a cancer indicator.

*5. Zinc/copper ratio of less than 4 parts of zinc to 1 part of copper . . . is a cancer indicator.

*6. Copper greater than 10 and less than 1.0 irregardless of ratio's . . . is a cancer indicator.

*7. Iron greater than 10 and less than 1.0 . . . is a cancer indicator.

Paul Eck believes that there are important interrelationships between minerals and vitamins. An excess of one mineral can cause an imbalance in another mineral in your body. Such imbalances can lead to illness. Here are some examples:

1. MANGANESE

Manganese can lower magnesium levels in the body. If your magnesium level is already low, the additional lowering by taking manganese can cause epileptic seizures and other neuro-muscular dysfunctions.

2. CALCIUM

Whenever you take large amounts of calcium, Eck states you will lose potassium. He says about 80% of the people in the United States suffer from a sluggish thyroid. This causes a high blood cholesterol, lack of incentive, fatigue. Eck says:

---

*These ratios figures are Paul Eck's testing figures. They are not standard ratio figures. What other testing laboratories for hair analysis may consider a normal ratio . . . Eck may consider not in the normal range.

> *Potassium is necessary for thyroxin, which is a hormone*
> *of the thyroid gland.*

Therefore, if one takes calcium causing a lowering in potassium
he will have a lowering of thryoid function.

Calcium will also drive magnesium out of the body causing a
high level of phosphorus to occur and make one prone to dental
cavities.

3. Vitamin B$_1$

   Large amounts of Vitamin B$_1$ can over a period of time cause
   a manganese deficiency. Initially, the taking of Vitamin B$_1$
   (thiamine) will give you a burst of energy. The excess of this B
   vitamin may also cause a magnesium deficiency. Both manganese
   and magnesium are important, Eck says, in blood sugar problems.
   Because of this manganese/magnesium dificiency, Eck believes,
   they can develop over 70 different diseases . . . including diabetes.

4. IRON

   Iron supplements can cause a copper deficiency. When too much
   iron is taken, Eck states, you can cause extremely high blood
   pressure, migraine headaches, and arthritis. Many arthritics have
   iron deposits in the joints of the body. Eck also reveals:

   > *Over 51% of all the cases of heart disease have been found*
   > *to have iron pigment deposits in the cardiac cells of the*
   > *heart . . . largely from taking too much iron or an inability*
   > *to properly metabolize iron.*[1]

   To give iron to raise iron is to lower iron. This is true of every
   mineral. When you have an iron deficiency, you give manganese.

5. ZINC

   Zinc supplements can cause a copper deficiency resulting in a
   severe anemia. By causing a copper deficiency the following
   conditions may result—menstrual problems, prostrate disorders,
   allergies, arthritis and insomnia to name a few.

6. COPPER supplements can over a period of time result in a
   Vitamin C deficiency. Excessive copper can also cause a Vitamin
   B-1 and B-6 deficiency.

---

[1]Ibid.

Impotency and frigidity problems are intimately associated with mineral ratio imbalances caused by "stress," diabetes, hypothyroidism, adrenal insufficiency, etc.

The **seven** main indicators, from a hair analysis, of impotence in a male or frigidity in the female are:

1. A 3.3 to 1 or less of calcium to magnesium level indicates that the individual has sexual problems of impotence or frigidity. This inverted ratio is found particularly in diabetics.
2. Sodium/Potassium inversion. The normal ratio is 2.5 of sodium to 1 of potassium. If this is inverted (less than 1.8/1), it is an indicator of sexual problems.
3. Copper. A very high copper level is another indicator.
4. Zinc. Extremely low or high zincs can also indicate sexual dysfunction and be a cause of impotence or frigidity.
5. A Sodium/Magnesium ratio greater than 18/1.
6. A Sodium/Zinc ratio greater than 8/1.
7. A Calcium/Sodium ratio greater than 10/1.

In the problems of obesity (overweight), Dr. Eck breaks down individuals into broad categories such as:

> Fast oxidation
> Slow oxidation
> Mixed oxidation

There are 3 different ways people metabolize their food. Dr. Eck refers to this as *Oxidation.* Oxidation is the use or burning of foods to produce energy on a cellular level. Regarding oxidation, Dr. Eck identifies the categories and suggests:

1. They are so fast
they are breaking down their sugars very rapidly and they have a great increase in heat production as a result. They are the type of people who, when they eat, they perspire a lot. They are *"fast oxidizers."* A *"fast oxidizer"* is a person who has a hyperactive thyroid and hyperactive adrenal glands. They tend to have excessive energy levels due to the fast burning of foods, followed by exhaustion.

2. They are so slow
that they are metabolizing their foods very slowly. They are *"slow oxidizers."* They have a hypoactive thyroid and hypoactive adrenal glands. Slow oxidizer's energy levels are usually low. This can be due to a number of factors such as the body's inability to completely break down the foods consumed when a HCl (Hydrochloric acid) deficiency is present. Low thyroid and adrenal activity also contributes to slow oxidation as well as toxic metal accumulation and dietary habits.

3. They are mixed oxidizers
who may be fast in one glandular area and slow in another. They tend to have energy swings as well as mood swings. This is due to the *"seesaw"* effect from fluctuating into fast and slow oxidation.

Both the fast and slow oxidizers are handling their foods the wrong way.

The Pill Destroys Sex Life Of Women

Dr. Eck believes that the Pill has destroyed the sex life of at least 10 million women.

The Pill creates a false pregnancy. The taking of a birth control pill raises the copper levels in the body. This creates a mineral imbalance which lowers your thyroid function as well as adrenal activity.

When a person has a low thyroid activity (hypothyroid), they don't have anywhere near the sex arousal . . . nor do they have a strong sex desire. They don't have the energy for it! Not only that, but the Pill brings with it menstrual period irregularities and menopausal disorders.

The male with high copper levels also develops a slow sexual arousal. Food that are high in copper include Brazil nuts, peanuts, sesame seeds, corn grits, broiled cod, baked flounder, broiled halibut, steamed lobster, pike and perch, ham, liver. Oysters are extremely high in copper. Just 1 cup of oysters (cooked, fried or raw) contains 59 milligrams of copper!

You also take copper into your body by drinking water coming through copper water pipes or cooking out of copper cookware.

Some women wear a copper IUD birth control device. Because the vagina is an acid medium ... that acidity leaches the copper off the coil and it goes into your system. Dr. Eck states that:

> It is estimated that there is enough copper
> eroded from a coil in one year
> to actually cause a person
> to become schizophrenic.[1]

In a pregnant woman, the copper keeps building up during pregnancy. The fetus stores a large amount of copper that he gets from his mother's liver. This usually last the child for 12 years.

> At the end of 12 years ... if the child's copper level
> does not go down ... you have females complaining of
> acne and adolescent problems, etc.

If the mother cannot quickly unload the copper excess after pregnancy ... she develops postpartum depression. Some women have become mentally unbalanced after giving birth. Paul Eck believes that copper excesses are the problem. Depending on the mineral imbalances of the individual, Eck uses either minerals or vitamins to unload the copper excesses. The hair analysis determines what supplements are needed.

What Results Can One Expect

Dr. Eck states that those who have a hair analysis and follow through on a personalized supplement program will experience symptomatic changes within two to three weeks. At least one year on supplements is needed to approach normalized mineral levels. Toxic metals and toxic minerals can be flushed out in about 6 months.

They may experience periodic worsening of their general condition depending upon their findings. As an example, if a person has rheumatoid arthritis, many times within the first two weeks there may be a marked reduction in pain. However, if the individual has

---

[1]Schizophrenia is *a major mental disorder typically characterized by a separation between the thought processes and the emotions ... a distortion of reality accompanied by delusions and hallucinations.*

numerous heavy metal accumulation, the removal from tissues and joints of these toxic metals will trigger a temporary flare-up in their condition. This may occur several times throughout the program. Dr. Eck suggests that if this flare-up of symptoms becomes too severe, the individual should reduce or stop taking his supplements for a few days until the symptoms subside.

Permanents, tints, bleaching and coloring of hair does not make any significant changes in hair analysis mineral readings. Some shampoos and hair treatments do affect mineral levels, however.

Selsun Blue may cause an elevation in selenium levels.
Head and Shoulders or Breck may result in elevated zinc.
Grecian Formula or other darkening agents will many times result in elevated lead levels. Lead acetate is used in these products to blacken the hair.

Dr. Eck suggests that hair analysis retests should be done three months after the first test to check progress. If the individual is a "mixed ozidizer" or "fast oxidizer," a retest is suggested in two months.

Dr. Eck says you cannot treat these people exactly the same as far as anything is concerned. You must take into consideration a broad classification of their oxidation types . . . preparing a program on that premise. You cannot give any one mineral for an obesity problem or any other problem. Hair analysis will determine what minerals are deficient and what minerals are in excess.

Paul Eck is very sold on proper hair analysis. In fact he is so sold on the necessity for hair analysis that he would not suggest any mode of treatment for any condition . . . to a physician . . . until a hair analysis of the patient has been made.

Hair analysis is becoming more and more popular. And there are quite a few hair analysis laboratories throughout the United States. Not all agree with Dr. Paul Eck's approach. In fact, he may be considered a maverick in the field. But his laboratory in Phoenix is kept very busy. It could be a sign that his customers are getting excellent results from his recommendations![1]

---

[1] Dr. Paul Eck, Analytical Research Labs, Inc., 2338 West Royal Palm Road, Suite F, Phoenix, Arizona 85021

FIGHTING CANCER WITH FOOD

FOODS

The Asparagus Diet

One biochemist, in a February, 1974 issue of *Prevention* magazine accumulated several case histories of those suffering from Hodgkins disease, bladder cancer and lung cancer. By adding asparagus to their diet, they experienced a return to normalcy. The biochemist added that asparagus should be cooked before eating.

SPROUTS

Inexpensive Insurance

As mentioned on Pages 80 and 81, sprouts are believed by many nutritionists to be an excellent insurance against Cancer as well as a healing agent for those with Cancer.

Alfalfa, lentils, mung beans and soy bean sprouts are among the most popular ones in use today. The Vitamin C content is five times higher in sprouts. Other vitamins increase in value as well.

In tests conducted by Charles R. Shaw, M.D., professor of biology at The University of Texas System Cancer Center in Houston ... it was discovered when test bacteria were exposed to the mutagenic substance in the presence of the extract from wheat grass sprouts, the mutation process was inhibited by up to 99%. Mung bean and lentil sprouts demonstrated a similar inhibitory effect.[1]

What this is saying is that the hereditary changes (mutation process) is repressed or restrained (inhibited). The theory that some nutritionists are working on is that the chlorophyll from these sprouts prevents formation of Cancer by restraining the enzymes which activate the carcinogens.

STARVING A TUMOR

Report on Melanoma

Malignant melanoma of the eye has regressed by dietary control ... according to a researcher in England. Writing in *Nutrition* (Vol. 28, No. 5, 1974), S. L. Stevens of Addenbrooke's Hospital, Cambridge, described the case of a 53-year-old chemistry teacher. He was diagnosed as having a large malignant melanoma of the left eye.

Surgery would have resulted in loss of all

[1]The Healing Force of Sprouts, (Emmaus, Pennsylvania: *Prevention*), March, 1979, pp. 133-137.

Many Nutritionists believe SPROUTS PROVIDE YOUR HIGHEST VITAMIN CONTENT Naturally!

Sprouts are actually described as *"perfect"* because all the life-giving proteins, carbohydrates, oils, vitamins and minerals necessary to support our life system are stored within the seed itself.

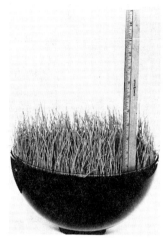

When seeds begin to sprout, their vitamin content accelerates at a remarkable rate. The first shoots of soybeans (per 100 grams of seed) contain about 100 milligrams of vitamin C, but after 72 hours the content soars to approximately 700 milligrams, an increase of almost 700 percent! **This means that soybean sprouts contain almost 20 times the amount of vitamin C that is provided in a glass of orange juice!** Similar comparisons can be made for most of the vitamins, including Vitamin A, the B vitamins and E.

Sprouts satisfy one's need for protein without consuming high calories. One ounce of meat, both lean and fat, contains approximately 80 calories ... whereas one ounce of beansprouts has only about 10 calories and ... contains no cholesterol!

There are some health clinics that specialize in "wheat grass therapy" in their approach to cancer patients. Many believe that sprouts are part of the answer to stopping the ravages of cancer and starting the healing process.

Sprouted seeds, the very beginning of new life, are one of the highest forms of nutrition known. They are free of chemical additives. You can grow them in your kitchen in just 12 inches of space! And you can have a harvest of nutritious home grown sprouts every 3 to 4 days.

There's a double bonus, too. Not only do you benefit by the nutritious value of sprouts, but you also save on your food bill.

**May
Help
Melanoma**

sight in this eye and vision in his right eye had been poor. Radiotherapy was out of the question because of the tumor's inaccessible location.

It was suggested that the patient try a low-phenylalanine, low-tyrosine diet. These are amino acids normally found in protein. The reasoning behind this is that limiting a diet to 10 grams of protein with low concentrates of these two amino acids . . . melanin systhesis is deprived of nutrients and the growth of melanoma is inhibited.

The patient was carefully monitored (because such regimin is walking a thin line bordering on malnutrition). However, the patient remained well and the malignant melanoma regressed when measured seven months later.

Can the lowly Asparagus cure cancer? No one knows. But there are some who do claim Asparagus has played a major role in healing them of cancer.

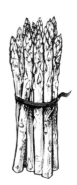

Asparagus is a part of the lily family. Asparagus is unusual, among our garden plants, in its flowering habits. While nearly all our vegetables bear both stamens and pistils (containing pollen cells and egg cells, respectively) on the same plant or in the same flower . . . Asparagus has two kinds of plants. About half bear only staminate flowers; the other half bear only pistillate flowers from which the little red seed-bearing fruits develop.

Asparagus was prized as a food by the Greeks and Romans and valued for the medicinal properties of all its parts. It has been cultivated in the Eastern Mediterranean and in Asia Minor for over 2000 years.

Before Asparagus was used for food, it had quite a reputation as a medicine for almost anything from the prevention of bee stings to heart trouble, edema *(abnormal accumulation of fluid in tissues)* and toothache.

Nearly all the green Asparagus is harvested with a little white on the butt end. Entirely green spears are cut at the surface and do not keep as well as those cut below the surface.

Here are some of the nutritive values in Asparagus:
Based on 4 spears/Canned, drained

18 Calories	42 Milligrams Phosphorus
2 Grams Protein	1.5 Milligrams Iron
3 Grams Carbohydrate	133 Milligrams Potassium
15 Milligrams Calcium	640 Milligrams Vitamin A
12 Milligrams Ascorbic Acid	

Asparagus provides an alkaline reaction in the body.

In 1975, William A. Ellis, D.O., made some interesting comments on the possible healing value of Asparagus. These remarks were recorded at an Endocrinology and Metabolism seminar in Sarasota, Florida.

His comments included the following:

> *Today, we are finding
> that almost all degenerative diseases
> have some form of microorganisms . . .*

He suggested one of the ways possibly to deal with this is to use Asparagus. The best Asparagus to use is the **canned** Asparagus . . . <u>not</u> frozen or fresh. He recommends Stokely or Jolly Green Giant varieties because they do not have pesticides or preservatives in the can.

Dr. Ellis suggests running the Asparagus through a blender to purée it. This transforms the Asparagus into a thick, moist, smooth-textured form.

> If one has Cancer, he suggests taking 4 tablespoons of this Asparagus purée with breakfast and 4 more tablespoons at supper. As a preventive he suggests 2 tablespoons in the morning and 2 tablespoons at supper. Dr. Ellis has found that this preventive program also aids diabetics and those with arthritis.

Dr. Jonas E. Miller of Sarasota, Florida related his experience with Asparagus at that same seminar. Dr. Miller had a first cousin living in Ohio who had an exploratory operation for cancer about 1975. She was told she could not live. Somewhere she heard of this Asparagus diet. As of 1981, his cousin has regained her health and is active.

One former patient of Dr. Miller had moved to the Midwest. During this time she developed cancer. Dr. Miller relates:

> When she came into my office, I was shocked.
> I hardly knew her. I said,
> *"What in the world is the matter with you?"*
> She replied that she had cancer.
> She brought her x-rays in
> and there was a mass
> almost as large as her head
> in her lung.

She told Dr. Miller that she was told she did not have long to live. But she heard about Asparagus and told Dr. Miller she was going to try it. Later, Dr. Miller checked her new x-rays and there was no evidence of the cancer mass. She became symptom-free.

Does the Asparagus therapy work? Only time will tell. One thing is certain . . . you will not experience harmful side effects from eating it!

THE HEALING POWER OF POSITIVE THINKING

MIND OVER CANCER

**Untapped
Resource**

Many believe that the brain is an untapped resource in the healing of Cancer.

Several reports conclude that one of the most consistent associations between psychological facts and Cancer is the loss of a major emotional relationship (such as a spouse) prior to the first symptoms of a disease.[1]

STRESS CAN BE A FRIEND OR FOE

**Stress
And
Cancer**

Since 1920, Dr. Hans Selye has been making a study of stress in its relation to disease. A stress rating scale, developed at the University of Washington is found on page 60 of the April, 1980 issue of *Prevention*. How a person handles stress can have a direct correlation to disease.

[1]A. Waller Hastings, Psychological Element of Cancer Tantalizes Physicians, *Family Practice News*, November 1, 1977, p. 12.

THE POWER OF POSITIVE THINKING

Mind Imagery

Carl Simonton, M.D. a specialist in oncology (the science of tumors) says results can sometimes be "truly amazing" when a Cancer patient allows his mind to participate in his treatment. He relates the story of a 61-year-old man with very extensive throat cancer who could barely swallow his own saliva.

> Dr. Simonton showed him
> . . . how through mental imagery,
> we were going to attempt
> to affect his disease.
> I had him relax three times a day,
> mentally picture his disease
> and his treatment
> and the way his body was interacting
> with the treatment and the disease,
> so that he could better understand his
>   disease
> and cooperate with what was going on.
> The results were truly amazing.[1]

Results Excellent

The man Dr. Simonton was treating had a complete remission. Prior to this "mental imagery" the patient had been depressed and sexually impotent for 20 years. The mental imagery program overcame his depression and restored his sexual prowess.

This "mental-visualization" of success is not a new discovery. Eugene P. Pendergrass, M.D., who was President of the

[1]Grace Halsell, Mind Over Cancer (Emmaus, Pennsylvania: Prevention), January, 1976, pp. 118-127.

American Cancer Society ... told the Society in 1960:

> There is solid evidence that the disease is affected
> by emotional distress ...
> It is my sincere hope
> that we can widen the quest
> to include the distinct possibility
> that within one's mind
> is a power capable of exerting forces
> that can either enhance or inhibit
> the progress of this disease.

A FUNNY THING HAPPENED TO ME ON THE WAY TO THE DOCTOR!

Laugh Your Troubles Away!

Back in 1970, J. I. Rodale wrote a book *Happy People Rarely Get Cancer*. More and more, those engaged in health are realizing that the mind plays an active part in accelerating or curing disease. You can have the best physician in the world, take the most complete combination of vitamins and minerals, stick to a highly nutritious diet ... and still die of Cancer! Why? Because if you have a negative, depressed and bitter attitude none of the popular health remedies may effect a cure.

The route to good health includes **(1)** Spirit, **(2)** Soul and **(3)** Body. They are interrelated ... and properly aligned, keep you in perfect harmony.

A Guide

In the Bible, in Proverbs 17:22 we read:

*A merry heart
doeth good like a medicine;
But a broken spirit
drieth the bones!*

This is good advice and it was written some 3000 years ago!

Is it possible to laugh your way back to vibrant health? Why not try it? It's free! There are no side effects! The only medicine that needs no prescription, has no unpleasant taste, and costs no money is laughter! So start laughing . . . right now! If you can't find anything to laugh about . . . just look in the mirror. You'll be hysterical!

1
VISUALIZATION THERAPY
A New Approach To Healing

Visualization therapy is so new that there are perhaps only a handful of doctors or health centers that practice it. It is being practiced with good success by a health center in California and in Wisconsin. This unusual therapy has proven very beneficial to those with cancer.

Visualization therapy is where the patient mentally visualizes his illness and also visualizes *"the forces of good"* attacking the illness and getting rid of it.

Doctors realize that the brain is an untapped resource in the healing process. Just now they are discovering the potential that the mind has over the body. This new energy of healing may become an important part of the overall approach to healing in the future.

In one example of visualization therapy, a Visualization Counsellor, Sheldon Rudeman, met with 7-year-old Michael Friedman. Michael had advanced kidney cancer.

> Michael visualized his cancer as an enemy invading his body. Part of this visualization therapy included drawing pictures of this *"monster"* trying to destroy his body.

Sheldon Rudeman asked Michael:

> How long will it take to get rid of this monster?

Michael replied:

> By the time I am 8.

At that time his eighth birthday was just 6 months away.

By age 11, Michael's cancer was in full remission. When asked how he *"destroyed"* the cancer monster, Michael replied:

> I shot it up with glue!

Sheldon Rudeman was a good Visualization Counsellor for he helped Michael acknowledge his illness and then by drawings and mind therapy visualize a positive all-out attack on this invading monster. Sheldon could counsel with compassion for he, himself had severe lung cancer. He was told he had two years to live. He used visualization therapy and six years later . . . was still alive.

Sara's Eye Healed

Sara was four and one-half years old . . . a healthy, normal child. But one day when she came home from play, her mother noticed that her left eye was red and swollen.

The eye became progressively worse. After three days, the left eye protruded almost three-quarters of an inch. She was taken to various prominent ophthalmologists and finally to an Eye Institute. Various medications were given her but were discontinued when hemorrhaging in the left eye occurred.

Various tests concluded that there were five blood tumors (*lymphangiomas*) behind the left eyeball. They were pressing on veins and the optic nerve, causing the protrusion. Sara's ability to see from this eye greatly deteriorated. The surgeons and ophthalmologists advised the parents that nothing could be done and stated that the eyeball would have to be removed.

Sara's parents fortunately attended a lecture on Wholistic Ophthalmology given by Leslie H. Salov, M.D. Dr. Salov is Director of the Vision and Health Center in Whitewater, Wisconsin.

Within a few days, Sara and her parents went to the center in Whitewater where therapy began. Dr. Salov explained to Sara in plain, simple language what her problem was.

> Sara spent her first day understanding her eye condition.
> That evening she drew a picture
> of what the back of her eye looked like.
>
> In her picture was her eye,
> with a face,
> the tumors,
> and a heart
> with the childish printing,
> I LOVE YOU,
>   Sara

At the next session, Dr. Salov explained to Sara what he terms: *"visual imagery."* He told her this would help her body to heal the eye. Dr. Salov relates:

> I explained to her that she was to look at the picture
> she had drawn of her eye,
>   with the five tumors behind it,
> and that as she did so,
> her mother would give her a pail
> and a small bulb filled with red water.
> As she squeezed the bulb,

she was to watch the red water flowing out,
and imagine that those tumors behind her left eye
were in the bulb;
that as she squeezed it
the bulb would be smaller and smaller
as the red water came out,
just like the tumors
behind her eyeball could.

Dr. Salov developed this concept when his own eyesight failed to the point of having to retire from practice. At first he could not accept this mode of treatment as scientific. But he was losing his vision due to macular degeneration. By using visual imagery he was successful in regaining 75% of his lost vision.

Dr. Salov also included color and light therapy in his healing techniques for Sara. Sara's room was painted a particular color of blue. She slept in a blue pup-tent and spent long hours outdoors with natural light bathing her face. All refined foods were eliminated and vitamin and mineral supplements added to her diet.

Dr. Salov first saw Sara in November. Within one month improvements in Sara's eye were noticeable. The eye returned to its normal orbital depth and the tumors were being absorbed. A year later, Sara's vision returned to almost normal. From a cosmetic viewpoint, she is already perfectly healed.

This heartwarming story is fully reported, along with comparative full color photographs in the June, 1981 issue of Let's Live magazine. The research interview is entitled Eyesight – A Barometer of Health and is written by Betty Lee Morales.

Light Can Affect Health

John Ott, a Florida researcher on the effects of light, discovered that fluorescent lighting was detrimental to good health. It is deficient in certain wavelengths. It is deficient in the blue spectrum area and also lacking in the invisible ultraviolet waves.

Qalbee Laird, M.D., director of a health center in Leicester, North Carolina, states:

Exposure to full-spectrum light
essentially increases our vitality.

The specific way it does that
is not yet known,
but it probably involves light's effect
on the pineal, pituitary and other glands,
and the hormones they secrete.

In addition,
light seems to increase
the body's protective immune response.[1]

Color Can Affect Health

A particular shade of pink can lower blood pressure, pulse and heart rate. This was reported in Biosocial: The Journal of Behavioral Ecology, November, 1980.

The effect of the pink color is physical, not psychological or cultural. Even people who are color-blind respond to its calming influence. Violent, aggressive inmates, when placed in a specially painted pink holding cell were calmed within minutes.

Sound Can Affect Health

Just as color and light can paint our moods, recharge our energies and aid in healing, so too can music (or sound).

Even the refrigerator's hum can become a source of family friction. It can increase the stress level in your life, reports sound researcher, Dr. Steven Halpern. The loud, rock-type discordant music that many teenagers listen to today could well be preparing them for serious illnesses in their 40's and 50's.

Your Subconscious And Your Health

Dr. Jonas Miller, a physician who practices in Sarasota, Florida is a firm believer in using the positive mental approach to healing. This approach is called Kinesiology.

It is a marriage of the relationship
of believing
and your subconscious.

---

[1]John Feltman, Healing With Light and Sound, (Emmaus, Pennsylvania: Prevention Magazine) June, 1981, p. 87.

What you put into your subconscious mind will affect every area of your life. If you allow negative or untruthful information to permeate your mind, Dr. Miller believes that it will definitely affect your daily life.

Dr. Miller has made a lifelong study of endocrinology . . . the study of glands. He states that the <u>thymus</u> gland serves as a monitor to your entire <u>nervous</u> and <u>muscular</u> system. These two systems are part of the <u>immune</u> system.

You are healthy . . . when your immune system is healthy. And you are more susceptible to disease . . . when your immune system is weakened.

Your thymus gland, then, is a key organism in triggering your immune system. Dr. Miller states:

> Rock music weakens a person
> while symphonic or religious music
> strengthens him.

He suggests a practical test to confirm this theory:

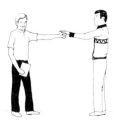

1. Extend your arm perpendicular from your body . . . at a right angle, parallel to the ground and make a fist.

2. While doing this, look at a pleasant picture cut out from a magazine (such as happy people or a country scene) and smile.

3. While doing this, have a friend simply apply about 10 pounds of pressure downward. Normally, you will be able to resist.

4. Now, remove the pleasant picture and replace it with a sad face or sad scene. Have your friend again apply about 10 pounds of pressure and you will find your arm has weakened. Why? Because your nervous and muscular systems have weakened as you look at the sad picture.

This test can also be used to check out such things as sugar, alcohol or tobacco. With your arm outstretched, if a teaspoon of sugar is placed on your tongue . . . your arm will weaken and will not hold up under applied pressure.

And simply looking at a cigarette or cigarette ad, Dr. Miller says, will automatically weaken your arm under pressure. Thus, negative forces of any kind will weaken you physically.

You Must Be Truthful

Dr. Miller relates a personal experience he had with a physician friend who had a very serious heart condition. This physician thought by telling himself he was actually getting better, that he would be healed. So he placed a tape recorder near his pillow at night and it kept repeating:

Every day in every way
my heart is getting stronger and stronger.

However, Dr. Miller says, his subconscious knew that his heart was not getting stronger and stronger and so it could not accept this information. It conflicted with the truth of the matter. One morning they found this doctor dead from a heart attack in his bed with the tape recorder going, *"Every day in every way my heart is getting stronger and stronger."*

When you place positive thoughts into your subconscious, they must be truthful. Dr. Miller says:

Never lie to your subconscious.
Don't say you're well when you're sick!
Don't say you're getting better
when you're not.

This is what the doctor was doing.
He was not acknowledging the sickness
and was trying to cover over a truth
his subconscious knew.
The result was conflict.
This was a form of double mindedness.

When you're saying you're getting better and better,
and it's true you actually are,
that's fine.

But if you're making this statement
and it's not true,
your subconscious knows you're lying
and won't follow through.

The Bible tells us to think on those things which are true, honest, just, pure, lovely and of good report. See Philippians 4:8 in the New Testament of the Bible. Perhaps one step to natural healing would be to stop watching the 6 o'clock news on television. Rarely does it have a *"good report."*

By channeling your mind on good things of a positive nature with your conscious mind, you reinforce your subconscious mind. This exercise begins to dispel the negative forces that create and sustain illness.

Picture Power Visualization

Dr. Miller believes that it is God's intention that man live a full life of 120 years. To augment this, he has placed around his bathroom medicine cabinet pictures of healthy people who are well over 100 years of age! By bathing his conscious and subconscious mind with this visualization of positive affirmation . . . he begins the day in the right spirit. We are reminded in the New Testament book of Ephesians in the Bible:

> . . . be renewed in the spirit of your mind.
>
> (Ephesians 4:23)

Living With A Healthy Attitude

In that same chapter (verses 31 and 32), we are reminded to eliminate from our life all bitterness, anger, quarreling, harsh words and dislike of others (malice). Instead, we are told to be kind one to another, tenderhearted, forgiving one another.

Dr. Miller suggests you monitor the way you speak. Start listening to the way you talk . . . about yourself, others and the world. Your speech will indicate the condition of your heart . . . not your physical heart . . . but your spirit.

> . . . out of the abundance of the heart
> the mouth speaketh.
>
> (Matthew 12:34)

Avoid negative statements. Instead of saying:

I have forgotten . . .

Be positive and channel into your subconscious the affirmation:

**I have trouble recalling,
but it will come to me shortly.**

Dr. Miller says that studies show that your mind is more efficient than a computer. Everything you have ever experienced in your life is not forgotten but stored in a memory bank.

To achieve good health, Dr. Miller states that the subconscious <u>cannot</u> deal in *"processes"* but only in completed concepts. Thus, to say:

I'm getting better and better . . .

is trying to feed a process to your subconscious. It cannot respond to a <u>process</u> . . . but only to a <u>completed</u> concept or picture.

If you are sick . . . you should repeat the phrase:

A normal, healthy body.

Your subconscious will accept this because it is a complete concept. You are not saying you have a normal, healthy body. You are merely expressing a truthful desire of your heart . . . which your subconscious can accept. Don't say you are well, when you are sick. But do visualize and say what you would like to become . . . a normal, healthy body.

Dr. Jonas Miller is not only a physician but an ordained minister. He relates the story of the time he was conducting a series of evangelistic meetings in a church in Alabama.

Separate Yourself From Your Sickness

A lady approached him who had a cancerous growth on her face. She told him:

I've got this cancer and I need prayer.

Dr. Miller told her to stop saying *"I've got this cancer,"* because:

. . . every time she was making this statement,
she claimed it as her own. I told her to
stop identifying with it.
It wasn't her cancer.
It wasn't God's cancer.

It was of the devil
>   and she should not lay claim to it
>   in any shape or form.

She went home and the next day came to the meeting wreathed in smiles. The cancer was no longer on her face. She told Dr. Miller she just stopped talking about her cancer. Instead she acknowledged that there was a cancer on her face, but it was not hers . . . it was the devil's.

What she did was acknowledge its existence, but she separated herself from the entire, negative, satanic thing and spoke positively through her faith in God, Dr. Miller reports.

She did not say she was well, when she was sick. But she separated herself from the sickness and refused to accept it as hers.

Dr. Miller says:

When you are sick, don't say, *"I'm well."*
Say *"good health"* or "a normal healthy body"
Keep it simple.
Keep it truthful and a completed concept.

Dr. Miller offers some advice in a humorous poem given him by a friend:

If you talk about your troubles
And tell them o'er and o'er
Then the world will think you like them
And proceed to give you more.

A complete review of Dr. Miller's concepts is found in his book: Prescription for Total Health and Longevity. It is written by Jonas Miller, M.D. with Jason Vinley and published by Logos International.

Laughter, light, sound, visualization therapy can become effective means of healing in your life.

Dr. Arnold A. Hutschnecker, in his book, The Will To Live wrote:
Depression
is a partial surrender to death.

Dr. Hutschnecker, an authority on psychosomatic medicine, believed that many diseases are nothing other than the expression of a person's need to withdraw, for a while, from the frays and strains of living.

Dr. O. Carl Simonton also believes that psychological forces play an important part in the development of cancer. He also believes that these psychological forces can be mobilized to defeat or delay its course. Dr. Simonton, in an article in <u>Health Action</u> (December, 1980), written by Maggie Scarf, reports that cancer flourishes in a climate of emotional despair.

One of the most effective ways of battling cancer, according to Dr. Simonton is by use of positive thinking through a technique he calls

<u>imaging.</u>

In this pattern of "imaging," cancer patients create mental images of a battleground. In this battle, the healthy cells are imagined chasing the malignant cells into a retreat.

Dr. Simonton is a physician who practices at:

Cancer Counseling and Research Center
6060 North Central Expressway
Suite 140
Dallas, Texas 75206
(214) 692-6311

Dr. Simonton has moved away from standard cancer therapy (chemotherapy and radiation) because he has found **healing through imagery** a better alternative. Dr. Simonton had skin cancer on his nose when he was 16. It took him a year to get rid of it.

Dr. Simonton believes that *"imaging"* which is supposed to influence the immune-defensive system can prolong life. Many patients in his program, according to Dr. Simonton, have approximately **twice** the normal life expectancy for their diagnoses. Criticism from medical colleagues almost drove him to leave the field of cancer medicine completely. They questioned his *"immune-defensive"* theory and stated that his theories were unproven.

However, Dr. Simonton, through his <u>Cancer Counseling and Research Center,</u> is actively pursuing his healing through imagery. Patients pay a fee of $1900 for a 10-day program. This includes group psycho-therapy sessions, psychological tests plus a physical examination.

Dr. William Donald Kelley is an orthodontist who became a nutrition consultant. He received his B.S., B.A., D.D.S. and M.S. from Baylor University in Texas. He then did postdoctoral work and completed his education towards his Ph.D. at Baylor University.

Dr. Kelley is the founder of the Council on Nutrition. He is a fellow of the International College of Applied Nutrition. He is also a member of the International Academy of Preventive Medicine.

He began his practice in orthodontics in 1954. By 1967 he was devoting full time to nutritional consultation. He has designed nutritional programs for about 8000 people . . . many in the celebrity status, including Steve McQueen, the late motion picture actor.

Dr. Kelley's views on cancer differ from the views of those in orthodox medicine. He states, in part:

> Basically, orthodox medicine
> has a fundamentally different approach
> to health than I do.
>
> Their approach is symptomatic.
> They don't treat the <u>disease</u> cancer –
> **the inadequate protein metabolism.**
> Rather, they treat the <u>symptom</u> of cancer –
> the tumor.
>
> But, you see, cancer is **NOT** a tumor.
> Cancer is a condition of
> inadequate protein metabolism.
> That's what gave rise to the tumor
> in the first place.
> Moreover, if not corrected,
> it will give rise to more tumors
> in the future, even if the
> first one is successfully removed.
>
> This, by the way, is the unfortunate
> reason why so many seemingly
> successful cancer operations
> end up in reoccurrences
> a year or two later.
>
> The tumor was removed, but the cause –
> improper protein metabolism –
> remained.[1]

---

[1] Sam Biser, <u>The William Donald Kelley Interview</u> (Charlottesville, Virginia: The Healthview Newsletter) 1978, Vol. 1, No. 5, p. 10.

Dr. Kelley defines cancer as

A trophoblast cell growing wildly in the wrong place.

It is the trophoblast cells which form the placenta. This anchors the newly formed embryo to the uterus. The trophoblast cell is one that invades other tissues. Kelley defines a link between cancer and a bodily imbalance. His program attempts to restore the proper balance.

Cancer has been described as *". . . another placenta, only out of place."* Women with cancer are sometimes suddenly cured when they become pregnant . . . yet for no apparent reason. The reason, Dr. Kelley believes, is that when the pancreas of the fetus is formed, it begins to secrete certain enzymes to stop the growth of the placenta. When these enzymes stop the placenta's growth . . . they stop the cancer also.

Dr. Kelley believes that the pancreas and its enzymes are the key to restoring a proper body balance. Kelley states that:

Cancer is simply the inability
to metabolize protein properly.

A pancreas
that cannot metabolize protein
cannot protect the body from cancer.

Based on Kelley's theory of cancer being the result of pancreatic malfunction, he notes that Diabetics have an abnormally high rate of cancer. The reason . . . because they have a diseased pancreas.

Kelley believes in most cases of pancreas impairment, the pancreas has been overworked by a diet too high in protein. A cancer patient cannot digest his food well because his supply of pancreatic enzymes is almost depleted. Kelley states:

Cancer kills its victims
by toxemia and starvation . . .
I've never seen a cancer victim
that didn't starve to death.[1]

Dr. Kelley believes that if a person with cancer has been told he has about 3 months to live . . . and decides to follow a well-designed nutritional program, he or she has a 60% chance of survival. Whereas, if a person has been told he has about 6 months to live . . . *"recovery should be almost routine."* Kelley optimistically feels

---

[1]Ibid., p. 4.

that almost all early cancer patients can be saved ... 98 out of 100. Kelley emphasizes that half-measures in following a nutritional program will not work for cancer patients. A strict nutritional program must be followed for success.

Kelley stated in his interview to The Healthview Newsletter that he has had good success with women with breast cancer.

Dr. Kelley does not accept any patient direct. The individual must first send for his "Request for Nutritional Consultation" form. The individual takes this form to his own doctor for his signature. This authorizes the nutritional program to begin.[1]

> A detailed questionnaire is sent.
> There are about 1000 questions to be answered.
> Your answers are analyzed by computer.

> An analysis is made of your current diet
> plus a new diet is formulated to match
> your particular body chemistry.

> Also included in the computer print-out
> is a recommended schedule of nutritional
> supplements, including enzymes, minerals and vitamins.

Dr. Kelley favors almonds. In fact, he calls his diet the almond diet and recommends them because they are an important source of protein. He suggests eating 10 almonds (no more, no less) along with breakfast and lunch. He also suggests a diet which includes raw seeds, alfalfa and mung bean sprouts, dry beans and eggs (soft boiled or raw).

He tells his patients to drink one pint of carrot juice every day. It is believed that the Vitamin A in the carrot juice helps destroy the protective coating on the cancer cells. This makes them more vulnerable to attack by pancreatic enzymes. His diet is one where 70% of the foods are raw.

SUPPLEMENTS

1. Kelley suggests that the most important supplement for cancer victims is a pancreatic enzyme supplement. His reason: *"this normalizes the protein metabolism and assists in devouring the cancer cells. No one in this society should eat protein without taking pancreatic enzymes at the same time. Pancreatic*

---

[1] The Kelley Program, Nutritional Counselling Service, 14455 Webb Chapel Road, Dallas, Texas 75234. Or call Toll Free 1-800 527-0227.

enzymes are the safest and cheapest insurance available against cancer, and they're tremendously effective."[1]

Dr. Kelley suggests 3 to 8 pancreatic enzyme tablets at each meal . . . each tablet to have at least 300 mg. of pancreas substance, or its equivalent which is 1200 mg. of pancreatin N.F.

> **2.** Kelley's <u>second</u> basic supplement is <u>blackstrap molasses</u> which he feels is an excellent source of minerals.

> **3.** He also recommends <u>hydrochloric acid tablets</u> as a <u>third</u> supplement to make sure the body absorbs the minerals properly.

> **4.** He includes in his diet a natural <u>multiple vitamin</u> supplement. He believes this is essential for cellular repair.

> **5.** Most everyone, Kelley believes, would benefit by taking a <u>comfrey-pepsin</u> supplement to get rid of the mucous coating in the small intestine. He suggests 2 capsules of comfrey-pepsin after each meal for one to three months. The pepsin is a digestive aid. The comfrey keeps the pepsin close to the intestinal wall so it can get at the detrimental mucus. For a person who has been ill, Dr. Kelley suggests that the comfrey-pepsin be taken for at least 6 months.

While Dr. Kelley favors avoiding meats, those who must eat meat . . . he suggests strongly that they eat it before 1 o'clock in the afternoon. He also suggests they take several enzyme tablets to digest these proteins.

Dr. Kelley uses 3 detoxification processes:

> 1. Coffee enemas
> 2. A purge and fast
> 3. A liver and gall bladder flush

A complete explanation of this is found in <u>The Healthview Newsletter</u>, Vol. 1, No. 5 (Box 6670), published in Charlottesville, Virginia 22906.

This Report is included for informational and educational purposes only. Neither Salem Kirban nor Salem Kirban, Inc. endorse or in any way recommend the advice given by Dr. Kelley or any other Report found in this book.

---

[1]Ibid., p. 5.

Bibliography
Recommended Reading

Airola, Paavo, O., *How To Get Well,* Health Plus Publishers, Phoenix, Arizona, 1976.

Atkins, Robert C., M.D., *Dr. Atkins' Nutrition Breakthrough,* William Morrow and Company, Inc., New York, 1981.

Brennan, Dr. Richard O., *Coronary? Cancer? God's Answer: Prevent It!,* Harvest House Publishers, Eugene, Oregon, 1979.

Bricklin, Mark, *The Practical Encyclopedia of Natural Healing,* Rodale Press, Emmaus, Pennsylvania, 1976.

Cooley, Donald G., *After-40 Health & Medical Guide,* Better Homes and Gardens Books, Des Moines, Iowa, 1980.

Donsbach, Jurt W., *Preventive Organic Medicine,* Keats Publishing, Inc., New Canaan, Connecticut, 1976.

Kirschmann, John D., *Nutrition Almanac,* McGraw-Hill Book Company, New York, 1975.

Mae, Eydie, *How I Conquered Cancer Naturally,* Harvest House Publishers, Eugene, Oregon, 1975.

Miller, Sigmund S., *Symptoms,* Avon Books, New York, 1976.

Nourse, Alan E., M.D., *Ladies' Home Journal Family Medical Guide,* Harper & Row, New York, 1973.

Null, Gary, *The Complete Question & Answer Book of Natural Therapy,* Dell Publishing Company, New York, 1972.

Nurse's Guide To Drugs, Intermed Communications, Inc., Springhouse, Pennsylvania, 1981.

Rodale, J.I., *Cancer Facts and Fallacies,* Rodale Press, Emmaus, Pennsylvania, 1969.

Rothenberg, Robert E., M.D., F.A.C.S., *The Complete Surgical Guide,* Weathervane Books, New York, 1974.

Medical Times, March, 1978, *(A Desk Reference Issue on Cancer),* Romaine Pierson Publishers, Inc., 80 Shore Road, Port Washington, Long Island, New York 11050.

Use this ORDER FORM to order additional copies of

The
MEDICAL Approach
Versus
NUTRITIONAL Approach
To
<u>CANCER</u>
by Salem Kirban

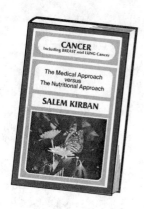

Your loved ones and friends will find
this book invaluable! Why not give this
excellent book to those who want honest answers to their problems.

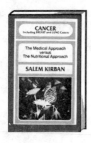

NOW! . . . You can make intelligent, life-changing decisions when you know **both approaches** to correcting ailments that plague you or your loved ones!

THE MEDICAL APPROACH
versus
THE NUTRITIONAL APPROACH

NEVER BEFORE . . . in one book . . . has an unbiased comparison been outlined, clearly, simply, showing both the Medical approach versus the Nutritional approach to major diseases!

At last! Sixteen books are now available! Each book defines the disease in words you can understand plus graphic pictures. The symptoms are also outlined.

Each book shows how medical doctors approach the examination of the patient, what tests they conduct, what drugs they recommend (and their side effects), the type of surgery followed and what their prediction is regarding the course of the disease and the probability of recovery (termed, *prognosis*).

In the same book, you will also read the Nutritional approach to the same disease; what natural therapy has been used through the years, what results have been achieved and what the prognosis is using nature's way.

Save by buying several books. Give to loved ones. You may be giving a gift of LIFE! **Each book is $5.**

The Medical Approach versus The Nutritional Approach

ARTHRITIS (including LUPUS)
by Salem Kirban

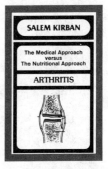

What causes arthritis? How many types of arthritis are there? Does medicine help or hinder? Is chiropractic treatment valid? How will the disease progress if not corrected? What do physicians recommend? What is the nutritional approach to the same problem? How is **Lupus** treated medically, nutritionally?

How to recognize the symptoms of arthritis. What diet do many nutritionists feel is beneficial? What foods should I avoid? Answers to these and more!

The Medical Approach versus The Nutritional Approach

CANCER
(including
Breast and Lung)
by Salem Kirban

What causes cancer? What do nutritionists believe is the cause of cancer? What are the basic types of cancer? Is surgery the answer? What about chemotherapy? Can drugs cure cancer? What side effects can I expect?

Is a proper nutrition program effective against cancer? What foods should I eat? Should I go on a juice diet?

The Medical Approach versus The Nutritional Approach

HEART DISEASE
by Salem Kirban

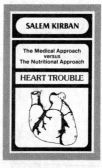

Does a diagnosis of heart trouble mean the end is near? Can I do something about it and live a happy, healthy long life . . . even after a heart attack?

What about drugs and Vitamin E? What is the sensible nutritional approach to the problem? How can I regain a sense of well-being and abundant energy without fear? What foods should I avoid? How can I flush my system clean again?

The Medical Approach versus The Nutritional Approach

HIGH BLOOD
PRESSURE
by Salem Kirban

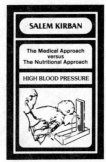

Why is high blood pressure dangerous? What are the causes? Is there any way nutritionally to lower my blood pressure? What drugs do medical doctors prescribe? What are the side effects? Do these "miracle" drugs really work?

What is the nutritional approach to high blood pressure? What juices should I drink? What vitamins and minerals are beneficial? Is fasting beneficial? What foods should I eat?

The Medical Approach versus The Nutritional Approach

DIABETES
by Salem Kirban ⑤

What causes diabetes? Must I change my lifestyle? Why do medical doctors prescribe insulin? What is the prognosis for one who is told he has diabetes?

Can a supervised nutrition program minimize the effect of diabetes? Will it provide a normal lifestyle? What foods should you eat? What juices are beneficial? Does the water I drink make a difference? Are vitamins and minerals and herbs worthwhile?

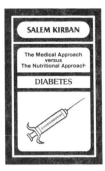

The Medical Approach versus The Nutritional Approach

BOWEL PROBLEMS
by Salem Kirban ⑥

How can I unlock my bowels for better health? How can I achieve that vibrant vitality again and gain that schoolgirl complexion? How can I break the laxative habit? Are drugs the answer?

How can I get rid of hemorrhoids forever? What vitamins and juices are especially beneficial? Are suppositories worthwhile? If so, what type? Can you have daily bowel movements and still be constipated?

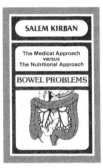

The Medical Approach versus The Nutritional Approach

PROSTATE PROBLEMS
by Salem Kirban ⑦

What are the early warning signs of prostate problems? What drugs do medical doctors recommend? What are the side effects? What surgery do they recommend? Is the cure worse than the problem?

Does the nutritional approach offer a more lasting alternative? What diet is recommended? How can you avoid prostate problems in sexual union? Why waiting to correct the problem is dangerous! Do juices and vitamins help?

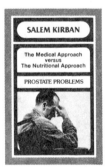

The Medical Approach versus The Nutritional Approach

ULCERS
by Salem Kirban ⑧

What causes gastric and duodenal ulcers? Are the "miracle" drugs really effective or do they bring with them a host of insidious side effects? What warning signals give you advance notice of an impending ulcer?

What foods are especially helpful? Are juices beneficial? Which ones and how should they be taken? What may happen if you don't change your way of life? What vitamins, minerals are beneficial?

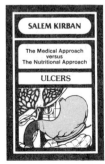

The Medical Approach versus The Nutritional Approach

KIDNEY DISEASE ⑨
by Salem Kirban

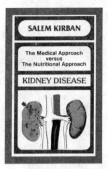

What is the medical approach to kidney disease? What are some of the problems that can develop if the disease is not nipped in the bud? What are the side effects of the drugs prescribed?

Is meat harmful? What type of diet is beneficial? Is a supervised fast recommended? How long? What common, ordinary foods and juices have proven beneficial? What vitamins and minerals help? What about herbs?

The Medical Approach versus The Nutritional Approach

EYESIGHT ⑩
by Salem Kirban

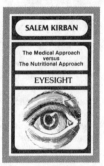

Are glasses the answer to failing eyesight? Is the medical approach to Cataracts the only solution? What do nutritionists recommend?

What eye exercises may prove beneficial for my eyes? Can I throw away my glasses? Is poor eyesight an indication of other growing physical problems? Can diet correct my poor eyesight? What juices may prove beneficial? What combination of vitamins and minerals should I take?

The Medical Approach versus The Nutritional Approach

IMPOTENCE/ FRIGIDITY ⑪
by Salem Kirban

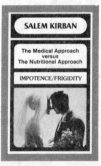

Impotence is the incapacity of the male to have sexual union. Frigidity is the incapacity of the female for sexual response. Both of these problems are growing because of today's stressful lifestyle! They lead to other trials!

What is the medical approach to these problems? How successful are they? What is the nutritional approach? What type of diet is recommended? Do juices help? Are herbs beneficial? Much more!

The Medical Approach versus The Nutritional Approach

COLITIS/CROHN'S DISEASE ⑫
by Salem Kirban

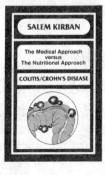

What causes Colitis? What drugs do doctors recommend? What are the side effects: How successful is surgery? What is the nutritional approach to Colitis? What foods are beneficial? What about juices and vitamins?

What is Crohn's Disease? What are the symptoms? Why does it recur? What is the medical approach to the problem? What is the nutritional approach? Can juices and vitamins correct the cause?

HOW TO BE YOUR AGAIN
HOW TO BE YOUNG AGAIN (13)
by Salem Kirban

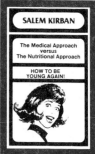

How can I restore my energy and eliminate fatigue? How can I develop Reserve Energy as an insurance to good health and a hedge against illness? How can I begin a simple, day by day health program?

How much should I eat and when should I eat? How can I check my own Nutrition Profile daily? How can I feel like 20 at age 60? How can I turn my marriage into a honeymoon again? When should I take vitamins, minerals? What juices are vital for a youthful life?

OBESITY (14)
by Salem Kirban

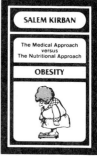

What causes Obesity? Why don't fad diets work? Is being overweight a glandular problem or a dietary problem? Is obesity a liver, pancreas or thyroid problem?

What is the medical approach to treating those who are overweight? What illnesses will obesity encourage? Why does the nutritionist treat your colon? What nutritional approach will take off weight easily and permanently giving you a new lease on life?

HEADACHES (15)
by Salem Kirban

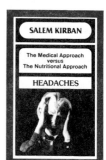

What causes headaches? Can headaches cause depression and hypoglycemia? Are women more prone to have nagging headaches? Must you live with migraine headaches all your life? What is the medical approach to headache problems?

Can a proper nutritional approach rid you of migraine headaches? Do vitamins help? Is fasting beneficial.? What about the pressure point techniques? What 3 herbs promise headache relief? How to tell your migraine *"Goodbye!"*

HYPOGLYCEMIA (16)
by Salem Kirban

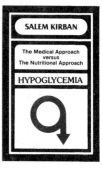

Is Hypoglycemia a fact or a fad? Why has this word . . . Hypoglycemia . . . become the focus of intense controversy? Is it the cause of many unexplained ills? What is the medical approach to this problem?

Anxiety, irritability, exhaustion, lack of sex drive, constant worrying, headaches, indecisiveness, insomnia, crying spells and forgetfulness . . . are these all signs of Hypoglycemia? How do nutritionists approach this problem with diet and supplements? Will this approach give you a new life?

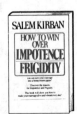

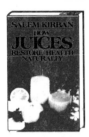
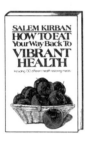
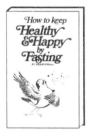
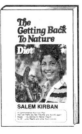

Quantity	Description	Price	Total
	The MEDICAL APPROACH Versus The NUTRITIONAL APPROACH Series		
_____	1 Arthritis	$ 5.00	_____
_____	2 Cancer	5.00	_____
_____	3 Heart Disease	5.00	_____
_____	4 High Blood Pressure	5.00	_____
_____	5 Diabetes	5.00	_____
_____	6 Bowel Problems	5.00	_____
_____	7 Prostate Problems	5.00	_____
_____	8 Ulcers	5.00	_____
_____	9 Kidney Disease	5.00	_____
_____	10 Eyesight	5.00	_____
_____	11 Impotence and Frigidity	5.00	_____
_____	12 Colitis/Crohn's Disease	5.00	_____
_____	13 How To Be Young Again	5.00	_____
_____	14 Obesity	5.00	_____
_____	15 Headaches	5.00	_____
_____	16 Hypoglycemia	5.00	_____
_____	**All 16 Health Books *(Save $30)***	**$50.00**	_____

Single Book	$5	All 16 Books	$50*
Any 3 Books	$12	(*You save $30)	

Other SALEM KIRBAN HEALTH BOOKS

_____	Unlocking Your Bowels For Better Health	4.95	_____
_____	How Juices Restore Health Naturally	4.95	_____
_____	How To Eat Your Way Back To Vibrant Health	4.95	_____
_____	How To Keep Healthy & Happy By Fasting	4.95	_____
_____	The Getting Back To Nature Diet	4.95	_____
_____	**How To Win Over IMPOTENCE/FRIGIDITY**	6.95	_____
	(Expanded Version with Full Color Section)		══════

Total for Books _____
Shipping & Handling _____
Total Enclosed $ _____

(We do NOT invoice. Check must accompany order, please.)

When using Credit Card, show number in space below.

☐ Check enclosed

☐ Master Charge   When Using MasterCard   Card | Month | Year
                    Also Give Interbank   Ex-
☐ VISA   No. (Just above your   pires
                    name on card)

*POSTAGE & HANDLING Use the easy chart to figure postage, shipping and handling charges. Send correct amount and avoid delay.

TOTAL FOR BOOKS	Up to 5.00	5.01-10.00	10.01-20.00	20.01-35.00	Over 35.00
DELIVERY CHARGE	1.50	2.00	2.50	2.95	NO CHARGE

FOR ADDITIONAL SAVINGS: Orders Over $35.00 Are Now Postage-Free!

SHIP TO _____
          Mr./Mrs./Miss   (Please PRINT)

Address _____

City _____ State _____ ZIP _____

SALEM KIRBAN, Inc./Kent Road, Huntingdon Valley, Pennsylvania 19006

FOR YOUR <u>LIFE</u> . . . KEEP INFORMED!

Now available! A quarterly Total Health Guide Newsletter to keep you up-to-date on the <u>very latest</u> of Medical/Nutritional Data! You owe it to yourself and to your loved ones . . . to be fully informed! Now! At last! You can have the <u>most current</u> information on diseases and their treatment . . . even before it is available to the general public! The information you receive may help save your life . . . or the life of a loved one!

<u>TWO</u> WAYS TO SUBSCRIBE

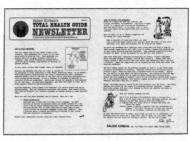

1. Total Health Guide Newsletter

Quarterly, for one year we will send you the 8-page Newsletter containing all the latest data on the major diseases. The Newsletter will present an unbiased report on both the Medical and Nutritional discoveries plus reports on their effectiveness and availability.

One Year: $25

2. Total Health Guide Newsletter
Plus

PERSONALIZED TYPEWRITTEN UPDATE

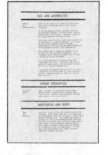

You will receive the quarterly 8-page Newsletter which reports the latest in Medical and Nutritional approaches to disease.

Plus! You will also receive a <u>TYPEWRITTEN REPORT</u> on the <u>specific disease in which you are personally interested.</u> This TYPEWRITTEN REPORT will be mailed to you within 3 weeks after you subscribe.

● You will also receive a <u>RING BINDER</u> to hold the Newsletters and Report. It will also contain a special unit to hold cassettes.

● Plus you will be sent the <u>cassette</u> . . .
  BALANCING YOUR EMOTIONS
  by Dr. Jonas Miller.

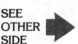

One Year: $50

SEE
OTHER
SIDE ➡

SALEM KIRBAN, Inc., Kent Road, Huntingdon Valley, Pennsylvania 19006

- -

YES! I want to keep informed! Send me the Health Information Service I have checked below. My check is enclosed.

☐ 1 Year / $25
   Total Health Newsletter

☐ 1 Year / $50 *(Fill in other side)*
   Total Health Newsletter
   Typewritten Health Report
   (Includes Ring Binder/Cassette)

Mr./Mrs./Miss   (Please PRINT)

Address

City   State   ZIP

REQUEST For Personalized TYPEWRITTEN HEALTH UPDATE

If you are subscribing for Medical/Nutritional Health Information for One Year at $50, you are entitled to a Typewritten Health Update on one disease.

It is important you understand that we neither diagnose or prescribe. Therefore we **cannot** make personal recommendations to you. Only your physician can do this. What we do provide you is the very latest in both Medical and Nutritional information on the disease in which you are interested.

Each month we go through hundreds of publications, books and listen to both medical and nutritional seminar cassettes. We cull from all of this the data that is essential to the particular disease in which you are interested.

We would be happy to answer specific questions in this TYPEWRITTEN HEALTH UPDATE providing they are not in the realm of diagnosing or prescribing.

DISEASE I want Data on_____

MY QUESTIONS I particularly would like answered: *(Please PRINT)*

1. _____

   _____

   _____

2. _____

   _____

   _____

3 _____

   _____

   _____

4. _____

   _____

   _____

**FILL IN
RESPONSE FORM
ON
REVERSE SIDE
AND
MAIL WITH YOUR CHECK**

ORDER FORM   SALEM KIRBAN Health Books

Quantity	Description	Price	Total
	The MEDICAL APPROACH Versus The NUTRITIONAL APPROACH Series		
_____	1 Arthritis	$ 5.00	_____
_____	2 Cancer	5.00	_____
_____	3 Heart Disease	5.00	_____
_____	4 High Blood Pressure	5.00	_____
_____	5 Diabetes	5.00	_____
_____	6 Bowel Problems	5.00	_____
_____	7 Prostate Problems	5.00	_____
_____	8 Ulcers	5.00	_____
_____	9 Kidney Disease	5.00	_____
_____	10 Eyesight	5.00	_____
_____	11 Impotence and Frigidity	5.00	_____
_____	12 Colitis/Crohn's Disease	5.00	_____
_____	13 How To Be Young Again	5.00	_____
_____	14 Obesity	5.00	_____
_____	15 Headaches	5.00	_____
_____	16 Hypoglycemia	5.00	_____
_____	**All 16 Health Books** *(Save $30)*	**$50.00**	_____

Single Book	$5	All 16 Books	$50*
Any 3 Books	$12	(*You save $30)	

Other SALEM KIRBAN HEALTH BOOKS

_____	Unlocking Your Bowels For Better Health	4.95	_____
_____	How Juices Restore Health Naturally	4.95	_____
_____	How To Eat Your Way Back To Vibrant Health	4.95	_____
_____	How To Keep Healthy & Happy By Fasting	4.95	_____
_____	The Getting Back To Nature Diet	4.95	_____
_____	**How To Win Over IMPOTENCE/FRIGIDITY**	6.95	_____
	(Expanded Version with Full Color Section)		

Total for Books _____
Shipping & Handling _____
Total Enclosed $ _____

(We do NOT invoice. Check must accompany order, please.)

When using Credit Card, show number in space below.

☐ Check enclosed
☐ Master Charge
☐ VISA

When Using MasterCard Also Give Interbank No. (Just above your name on card)

Card | Month | Year
Expires

*POSTAGE & HANDLING Use the easy chart to figure postage, shipping and handling charges. Send correct amount and avoid delay.

TOTAL FOR BOOKS	Up to 5.00	5.01-10.00	10.01-20.00	20.01-35.00	Over 35.00
DELIVERY CHARGE	1.50	2.00	2.50	2.95	NO CHARGE

FOR ADDITIONAL SAVINGS: Orders Over $35.00 Are Now Postage-Free!

SHIP TO _____
Mr./Mrs./Miss   (Please PRINT)

Address _____

City _____ State _____ ZIP _____

SALEM KIRBAN, Inc./Kent Road, Huntingdon Valley, Pennsylvania 19006

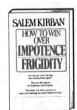

ORDER FORM   **SALEM KIRBAN Health Books**

Quantity	Description	Price	Total
	The MEDICAL APPROACH Versus The NUTRITIONAL APPROACH Series		
_____	1 Arthritis	$ 5.00	_____
_____	2 Cancer	5.00	_____
_____	3 Heart Disease	5.00	_____
_____	4 High Blood Pressure	5.00	_____
_____	5 Diabetes	5.00	_____
_____	6 Bowel Problems	5.00	_____
_____	7 Prostate Problems	5.00	_____
_____	8 Ulcers	5.00	_____
_____	9 Kidney Disease	5.00	_____
_____	10 Eyesight	5.00	_____
_____	11 Impotence and Frigidity	5.00	_____
_____	12 Colitis/Crohn's Disease	5.00	_____
_____	13 How To Be Young Again	5.00	_____
_____	14 Obesity	5.00	_____
_____	15 Headaches	5.00	_____
_____	16 Hypoglycemia	5.00	_____
_____	**All 16 Health Books (Save $30)**	**$50.00**	_____

Single Book	$5	All 16 Books	$50*
Any 3 Books	$12	(*You save $30)	

Other SALEM KIRBAN HEALTH BOOKS

_____	Unlocking Your Bowels For Better Health	4.95	_____
_____	How Juices Restore Health Naturally	4.95	_____
_____	How To Eat Your Way Back To Vibrant Health	4.95	_____
_____	How To Keep Healthy & Happy By Fasting	4.95	_____
_____	The Getting Back To Nature Diet	4.95	_____
_____	**How To Win Over IMPOTENCE/FRIGIDITY**	6.95	_____
	(Expanded Version with Full Color Section)		

Total for Books _____
Shipping & Handling _____
Total Enclosed $

(We do NOT invoice. Check must accompany order, please.)

When using Credit Card, show number in space below.

☐ Check enclosed

☐ Master Charge

☐ VISA

When Using MasterCard
Also Give Interbank
No. (Just above your
name on card)

Card	Month	Year
Ex-pires		

POSTAGE & HANDLING Use the easy chart to figure postage, shipping and handling charges. Send correct amount and avoid delay.

TOTAL FOR BOOKS	Up to 5.00	5.01-10.00	10.01-20.00	20.01-35.00	Over 35.00
DELIVERY CHARGE	1.50	2.00	2.50	2.95	NO CHARGE

FOR ADDITIONAL SAVINGS: Orders Over $35.00 Are Now Postage-Free!

SHIP TO _____
          Mr./Mrs./Miss   (Please PRINT)

Address _____

City _____ State _____ ZIP _____

SALEM KIRBAN, Inc./Kent Road, Huntingdon Valley, Pennsylvania 19006